INTERVENTIONAL CARDIOLOGY CLINICS

www.interventional.theclinics.com

Editor-in-Chief

MATTHEW J. PRICE

Transcatheter Closure of Patent Foramen Ovale

October 2017 • Volume 6 • Number 4

Editor

MATTHEW J. PRICE

ELSEVIER

1600 John F. Kennedy Boulevard • Suite 1800 • Philadelphia, Pennsylvania, 19103-2899

http://www.theclinics.com

INTERVENTIONAL CARDIOLOGY CLINICS Volume 6, Number 4
October 2017 ISSN 2211-7458, ISBN-13: 978-0-323-54670-6

Editor: Lauren Boyle
Developmental Editor: Donald Mumford

Interventional Cardiology Clinics (ISSN 2211-7458) is published quarterly by Elsevier Inc., 360 Park Avenue South, New York, NY 10010-1710. Months of issue are January, April, July, and October. Subscription prices are USD 195 per year for US individuals, USD 449 for US institutions, USD 100 per year for US students, USD 195 per year for Canadian individuals, USD 536 for Canadian institutions, USD 150 per year for Canadian students, USD 295 per year for international individuals, USD 536 for international institutions, and USD 150 per year for international students. To receive student/resident rate, orders must be accompanied by name of affiliated institution, date of term, and the *signature* of program/residency coordinator on institution letterhead. Orders will be billed at individual rate until proof of status is received. Foreign air speed delivery is included in all *Clinics* subscription prices. All prices are subject to change without notice. **POSTMASTER:** Send address changes to *Interventional Cardiology Clinics*, Elsevier Health Sciences Division, Subscription Customer Service, 3251 Riverport Lane, Maryland Heights, MO 63043. **Customer Service: Telephone: 1-800-654-2452** (U.S. and Canada); **1-314-447-8871** (outside U.S. and Canada). **Fax: 1-314-447-8029. E-mail: journalscustomerservice-usa@elsevier.com (for print support); journalsonlinesupport-usa@elsevier.com (for online support).**

Reprints. For copies of 100 or more of articles in this publication, please contact the Commercial Reprints Department, Elsevier Inc., 360 Park Avenue South, New York, NY 10010-1710. Tel.: 212-633-3874; Fax: 212-633-3820; E-mail: reprints@elsevier.com.

CONTRIBUTORS

EDITOR-IN-CHIEF

MATTHEW J. PRICE, MD
Director, Cardiac Catheterization Laboratory, Division of Cardiovascular Diseases, Scripps Clinic, Assistant Professor, Scripps Translational Science Institute, La Jolla, California, USA

EDITOR

MATTHEW J. PRICE, MD
Director, Cardiac Catheterization Laboratory, Division of Cardiovascular Diseases, Scripps Clinic, Assistant Professor, Scripps Translational Science Institute, La Jolla, California, USA

AUTHORS

ISLAM ABUDAYYEH, MD
Assistant Professor of Medicine, Division of Cardiology, Interventional Cardiology, Loma Linda University Health, Loma Linda, California, USA

NAYAN AGARWAL, MD
Cardiology Fellow, Division of Cardiology, Department of Medicine, University of Florida, Gainesville, Florida, USA

MARY Z. BECHIS, MD
Cardiac Non-Invasive Laboratory, Division of Cardiovascular Diseases, Scripps Clinic, La Jolla, California, USA

ISLAM Y. ELGENDY, MD
Cardiology Fellow, Division of Cardiology, Department of Medicine, University of Florida, Gainesville, Florida, USA

DAVID HILDICK-SMITH, MD, BM, BChir
Sussex Cardiac Centre, Brighton and Sussex University Hospitals, Brighton, United Kingdom

AHMED N. MAHMOUD, MD
Cardiology Fellow, Division of Cardiology, Department of Medicine, University of Florida, Gainesville, Florida, USA

EMILIYA MELKUMOVA, MD
Vascular and General Neurologist, Associate Program Director of Tufts Neurology Residency Program, Department of Neurology, Tufts Medical Center, Assistant Professor of Neurology, Tufts University School of Medicine, Boston, Massachusetts, USA

MOHAMMAD KHALID MOJADIDI, MD
Cardiology Fellow, Division of Cardiology, Department of Medicine, University of Florida, Gainesville, Florida, USA

DEEPIKA NARASIMHA, MD
Division of Cardiology, Interventional Cardiology, Loma Linda University Health, Loma Linda, California, USA

OLUFUNSO W. ODUNUKAN, MBBS, MPH
Division of Cardiovascular Diseases, Scripps Clinic, La Jolla, California, USA

MATTHEW J. PRICE, MD
Director, Cardiac Catheterization Laboratory, Division of Cardiovascular Diseases, Scripps Clinic, Assistant Professor, Scripps Translational Science Institute, La Jolla, California, USA

DAVID S. RUBENSON, MD
Director, Cardiac Non-Invasive Laboratory,
Division of Cardiovascular Diseases, Scripps
Clinic, La Jolla, California, USA

DAVID E. THALER, MD, PhD, FAHA
Chairman, Department of Neurology, Director
Emeritus, Comprehensive Stroke Center, Tufts
Medical Center, Professor of Neurology, Tufts
University School of Medicine, Boston,
Massachusetts, USA

JONATHAN M. TOBIS, MD, FACC, MSCAI
Emeritus Director of Interventional Cardiology
Research, Professor of Medicine, Division of
Cardiology, Department of Medicine, David
Geffen School of Medicine at UCLA, Los
Angeles, California, USA

TIMOTHY M. WILLIAMS, BA, BM, BCh
Sussex Cardiac Centre, Brighton and Sussex
University Hospitals, Brighton, United
Kingdom

CONTENTS

Stroke is a devastating condition. It is the fifth leading cause of death in the United States, and a leading cause of serious long-term disability. Stroke occurs at any age. Younger patients tend to have strokes of undetermined cause, termed cryptogenic. Herein, the authors describe the classification of stroke cause; the risk of recurrent cryptogenic stroke with patent foramen ovale (PFO); a risk assessment model to stratify incidental versus a pathogenic PFO in patients presenting with stroke; and patient selection for device occluder therapy in the context of the long-term follow-up of the RESPECT randomized clinical trial.

Once deemed benign, patent foramen ovale (PFO)–mediated right-to-left shunting has now been linked to stroke, migraine, and hypoxemia. Contrast transesophageal echocardiography is considered the standard technique for identifying a PFO, allowing visualization of the atrial septal anatomy and differentiation from non-PFO right-to-left shunts. Transthoracic echocardiography is the most common method for PFO imaging, being cost-effective, but has the lowest sensitivity. Transcranial Doppler is highly sensitive but is unable to differentiate cardiac from pulmonary shunts; it is the best method to quantitate shunt severity, being more sensitive than transthoracic or transesophageal echocardiography, thus is the authors' preferred screening method.

Transcatheter closure of atrial septal defects and patent foramen ovale has become increasingly common with advances in device and imaging technology. The percutaneous approach is now the preferred method of closure when anatomically suitable. Two-dimensional and 3-dimensional echocardiography determines anatomic suitability by characterizing the interatrial defect and its surrounding structures and is critical for intraprocedural guidance and postprocedure follow-up. This article provides an overview of interatrial anatomy as it pertains to interventional considerations and discusses the transthoracic, transesophageal, and intracardiac echocardiographic modalities used for periprocedural and intraprocedural imaging of the interatrial septum.

Approximately one-third of all strokes have no apparent cause. A patent foramen ovale (PFO) is present in as many as 60% of these patients with cryptogenic strokes, which is significantly more frequent than that of the general
population. The presumed biologic mechanisms of ischemic stroke in the
setting of a PFO are paradoxic embolism from the peripheral venous system
through this interatrial shunt or embolism from in situ thrombosis. In this review, the authors summarize and critically assess the contemporary studies
evaluating the efficacy and safety of PFO closure for prevention of recurrent
cryptogenic strokes.

Migraine headache is a common and debilitating disease that has a demon-
strable association with the presence of patent foramen ovale (PFO) in multiple
case series. Closure of PFO has been performed to try to treat migraine with
aura, with variable results. Although early trials suggested benefit to PFO
closure, these were of poor quality, and subsequent randomized trials have
failed to yield positive results. This article discusses the evidence of an association with PFO and migraine headache, and the trials that have so far been performed to assess the benefits of closure.

A patent foramen ovale (PFO) is a common anatomic finding in 20% of the
normal population. Significant hypoxemia can occur in circumstances in which
hemodynamic or anatomic changes predispose to increased right-to-left intra-
atrial shunting. The subsequent hypoxemia produces substantial dyspnea that
may affect the patient's quality of life, independent of underlying pulmonary
disease. Profound hypoxemia caused by right-to-left shunt across the interatrial
septum usually responds to percutaneous PFO closure. An important impediment to successful treatment is the lack of awareness of the potential role of a
PFO in this condition.

Transcatheter closure of a patent foramen ovale (PFO) reduces the risk of recurrent cryptogenic stroke compared with medical therapy. PFO closure is a prophylactic procedure and will not provide the patient with symptomatic
improvement, except in cases of hypoxemia due to right-to-left shunt or
possibly migraine headaches. Therefore, appropriate patient selection is critical, and procedural safety is paramount. Herein, the authors review key characteristics of the devices currently available for transcatheter PFO closure
within the United States and highlight key technical aspects of the PFO closure
procedure that will maximize procedural success.

TRANSCATHETER CLOSURE OF PATENT FORAMEN OVALE

THE CLINICS ARE NOW AVAILABLE ONLINE!

Access your subscription at:
www.theclinics.com

PREFACE

Transcatheter Closure of Patent Foramen Ovale

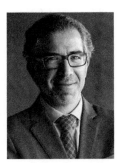

Matthew J. Price, MD
Editor

A patent foramen ovale (PFO) is a common anatomic finding that occurs in approximately one-quarter of the population. The presence of a PFO has been linked to a host of pathologic conditions, including but not limited to cryptogenic stroke, migraine headache with aura, and hypoxemia due to right-to-left shunt. In late 2016, the US Food and Drug Administration (FDA) approved transcatheter PFO closure with the Amplatzer PFO Occluder (St Jude, St. Paul, MN, USA) to reduce the risk of recurrent cryptogenic stroke. The path to approval has been long and arduous. Devices for PFO closure were introduced more than a decade ago under a Humanitarian Device Exemption (HDE) in the absence of data for clinical efficacy. However, the exuberant adoption of this therapy by interventional cardiologists led the FDA to suspend the HDE. Similar or identical devices had been approved or cleared for transcatheter closure of atrial septal defects, resulting in a dilemma for clinical researchers and clinicians: randomized clinical trials to prove the safety and efficacy of transcatheter PFO closure compared with medical therapy

were enrolling at the same time that the devices were commercially available (albeit off-label). As a result, the clinical trials were very slow to enroll, and there was likely bias to enroll the lowest-risk patients, as clinicians would be more likely to treat those they considered at highest risk with device closure in an off-label fashion, rather than enroll them in a clinical trial in which they could be randomly assigned to medical therapy. In addition, the efficacy of PFO closure might only be seen after a prolonged duration of follow-up, given the low absolute yearly risk of thromboembolic events in younger patients with cryptogenic stroke. The neutral outcomes of flawed trials with relatively short-term follow-up, composite endpoints, and possibly too broad enrollment criteria put transcatheter PFO closure out to pasture, far from the focus of the interventional and neurologic community.

However, more than a decade later, PFO closure is now again front and center for cryptogenic stroke treatment, as the long-term outcomes of the RESPECT trial demonstrated that transcatheter closure is an effective treatment

Intervent Cardiol Clin 6 (2017) ix–x
http://dx.doi.org/10.1016/j.iccl.2017.07.001
2211-7458/17/© 2017 Published by Elsevier Inc.

option for patients with a PFO and imaging-documented stroke from an unknown cause. When treating patients, the interventional cardiologist will be confronted with a panoply of issues, such as the required workup for ischemic stroke; how to image and evaluate PFO anatomy; assessment of stroke risk based on clinical and anatomic factors; appropriate patient selection; device choice and implantation technique; and the role of transcatheter PFO closure in a range of other clinical conditions. This issue of *Interventional Cardiology Clinics* will therefore serve the reader well, as it represents the current state-of-the art for PFO diagnosis, assessment, and percutaneous management from the perspective of world leaders in the field.

Matthew J. Price, MD
Cardiac Catheterization Laboratory
Division of Cardiovascular Diseases
Scripps Clinic
Scripps Translational Science Institute
9898 Genesee Avenue
Suite AMP-200
La Jolla, CA 92037, USA

E-mail address:
price.matthew@scrippshealth.org

Cryptogenic Stroke and Patent Foramen Ovale Risk Assessment

Emiliya Melkumova, MD*, David E. Thaler, MD, PhD

KEYWORDS

- Cryptogenic stroke • Embolic stroke of undetermined source • Patent foramen ovale (PFO)
- Selecting patients for PFO closure • Recurrent embolic stroke • Secondary stroke prevention
- Risk of paradoxic embolism (RoPE) score • Stroke in young adults

---

KEY POINTS

- Individualized comprehensive investigations are required for patients with embolic ischemic stroke before being labeled cryptogenic. There is no gold standard.
- Not all discovered patent foramen ovales (PFOs) in cryptogenic stroke patients are pathogenic.
- Because PFO-related embolic strokes tend to affect young adults, the cumulative risk of recurrence is substantial even though there is a relatively low annual incidence of recurrence.
- PFO closure should only be expected to prevent PFO-related stroke recurrences.
- The RoPE score is a tool that may be used to determine the likelihood that the index stroke is causally related to the detected PFO.

INTRODUCTION

Stroke is the fifth leading cause of death in the United States, and the second leading cause of death globally.[1] Cryptogenic stroke is a diagnosis of exclusion that assumes that appropriate investigations have been conducted to identify other plausible and relevant causes, but none have been found. The foramen ovale is a small, flaplike opening between the right and the left atria that permits right-to-left intracardiac shunting in the developing fetus. It remains patent beyond the first few months of life, without complete closure, in about 25% of the general population.[2–4] The patent foramen ovale (PFO) may act as a nidus for clot formation or as a conduit through which a thrombus can travel, thereby bypassing the natural filtration provided by the capillaries in the lungs. Paradoxic embolism refers to the paradox of a venous source thrombus appearing in the arterial circulation without being filtered out in the pulmonary circulation. Paradoxic embolism is a widely accepted mechanism of stroke. However, in the absence of direct visualization of a thrombus in the PFO itself, the diagnosis is still "presumed" in the setting of an otherwise cryptogenic stroke. The currently accepted terminology is cryptogenic stroke with PFO. Herein, the authors describe the classification of stroke cause; the risk of recurrent cryptogenic stroke with PFO; a risk assessment model to stratify incidental versus a pathogenic PFO in patients presenting with stroke; and patient selection for device occluder therapy in the context of the recent US Food and Drug Administration (FDA) approval of transcatheter PFO closure.

Disclosure Statement: Dr E. Melkumova has no financial disclosures or conflicts of interest related to this article. Dr D.E. Thaler reports being a consultant to Abbott (Steering Committee, RESPECT Trial) and receiving grant funding from NINDS for the RoPE Study (R01 NS062153).

Department of Neurology, The Comprehensive Stroke Center, Tufts Medical Center, Tufts University School of Medicine, 800 Washington Street, Box 314, Boston, MA 02111, USA

* Corresponding author.

E-mail address: emelkumova@tuftsmedicalcenter.org

STROKE NOMENCLATURE AND CLASSIFICATION

Stroke is an observation, not a diagnosis. It is a compilation of signs and symptoms. There are typical and atypical stroke-like presentations, and therefore, neurologic expertise is required to accurately differentiate between strokes, stroke mimics, stroke-like chameleons, and non-stroke presentations. *True strokes* are strokes with typical presentations; *stroke-chameleons* are strokes with atypical presentations that are initially interpreted as non-strokes; *stroke-mimics* are spells with typical stroke-like presentations, but are not strokes; and *non-strokes* are spells with atypical stroke-like presentations and are indeed not strokes. The stroke-chameleons and the stroke-mimics are particularly challenging, because their clinical presentations are typically misleading, hence the names. Boxes 1 and 2 provide partial examples of stroke mimics and stroke chameleons, respectively.[5–7] According to one retrospective chart review, the common stroke-chameleons were admitted under misdiagnoses of altered mental status (30.9%), syncope (16.0%), hypertensive emergency (12.8%), systemic infection (10.6%), suspected acute coronary syndrome (9.6%), and other (20.1%).[7] Misdiagnosis has significant implications for stroke therapy, patient outcome, and prognosis.

The common mechanisms for true stroke include small-vessel disease (ie, lipohyalinosis and atherosclerosis), embolism, and rarely, decreased perfusion through a fixed stenosis. Some of the less common, but equally important, mechanisms for stroke are listed in Box 3. Emboli can be broken down further into those that arise from other arteries, those that arise from the heart, or those that paradoxically start in the venous system but which gain access to the arteries via a right-to-left shunt.

A true culprit is not identified for many patients with stroke despite thorough investigations for a cause. Their strokes are labeled cryptogenic (*crypto* from the Greek for "hidden" and *genesis* for "source"). Cryptogenic stroke is a diagnosis of exclusion that assumes that investigations have been conducted to identify other plausible and relevant causes.[8] There is no gold-standard study or battery of tests. Each patient's unique characteristics demand a thoughtful approach to stroke evaluation. Our genetic composition, environmental influences, and lifestyle choices mold us into who we are and lead to the variability in our individual cerebrovascular risk factors. Different classification schemes have attempted to define strokes by etiologic subtypes. Commonly used schemes include the Trial of ORG-10172 in Acute Stroke Treatment (TOAST) classification, the CCS (Causative Classification Scheme), and ASCOD (Atherosclerosis, Small-vessel disease, Cardiac causes, Other, and Dissection). These classification schemes were originally developed for research but have made their way into clinical practice. The TOAST criteria have been particularly dominant.

The term *cryptogenic stroke* is used loosely to describe 4 categories of stroke patients: *undermeasured, underclassified, competing causes,* and *true cryptogenic stroke.* Undermeasured patients have not yet undergone a thorough

---

Box 2
Stroke chameleons

Neuropsychiatric symptoms

Abnormal movements or seizures

Peripheral nervous system symptoms

Isolated dysarthria

Localized asterixis

Cortical blindness with denial of deficit

Acute monoparesis

Negative MRI in acute ischemic stroke

Box 1
Stroke mimics

Alcohol intoxication

Migraine

Epilepsy

Brain tumor

Brain abscess

Hypoglycemia or hyperglycemia

Peripheral vertigo

Encephalitis

Box 3
Uncommon causes of cerebral ischemia

Arterial dissection

Hypercoagulable states

Vasospasm

Vasculitis

Collagen vascular diseases

Meningitis

Hematologic disorders

Intracranial venous thrombosis

diagnostic investigation, and therefore, the causality of stroke in this group is uncertain. Underclassified patients have a suspected culprit identified, but that culprit does not meet standardized criteria for causality to be assigned. In patients with competing causes, there are multiple potential causes that meet the standardized criteria for causality, for example, atrial fibrillation in the presence of a high-grade ipsilateral carotid stenosis, and so deciding among them is impossible. True cryptogenic strokes are those in which adequate and extensive diagnostic evaluations are "normal," that is, these evaluations do not suggest a potential cause.[9] Among populations of stroke patients, the prevalence of true cryptogenic stroke is 15% to 35%.[10]

The 5-year risk of stroke recurrence from all causes is approximately 20%; hence, timely index stroke diagnosis and secondary stroke prevention are crucial.[1] Modification of vascular risk factors along with antiplatelet therapy and high-dose statin therapy play a role in preventing strokes, from small-vessel disease, branch disease, aortic arch atheroma, and artery-to-artery embolization. Anticoagulation therapy is used for cardioembolic stroke prevention in patients with atrial fibrillation, left ventricular regional wall akinesis, and very low ejection fractions. Management of cerebral venous thrombosis requires anticoagulation even in the setting of acute hemorrhage. The optimal medical management of PFO-related stroke remains uncertain, but it involves a combination of an antithrombotic agent and percutaneous transcatheter closure device in select patients.

RISK OF PARADOXIC EMBOLISM SCORE
Patent Foramen Ovale–Attributable Risk
A review of 23 case-control studies found that the prevalence of PFO among cryptogenic stroke patients (40%) is higher than in the general population (25%).[11] The overrepresentation among cryptogenic stroke patients argues strongly for an association between PFO and stroke. The physiology of paradoxic embolism is understood, and so the epidemiologic association can be presumed to be causal. However, given the high prevalence in the general population, it is likely that up to half of all discovered PFOs in cryptogenic stroke patients are incidental and were not related to the index event. Therefore, it is important to determine the infarct mechanism, because not all discovered PFOs in cryptogenic stroke patients are pathogenic. A goal of the Risk of Paradoxic Embolism (RoPE) study was to disaggregate discovered PFOs in cryptogenic stroke patients into those that are likely to have

been pathogenic (and so may need treatment) from those that are likely to be incidental (and so potentially ignorable).

The RoPE study produced a means by which individual patients could be offered a probability that their discovered PFO was or was not related to their stroke.[12] The RoPE score can be calculated based on easily obtainable variables available at the time of the index event (**Box 4**).[13] The range of RoPE scores is 0 to 10. The maximum score of 10 is given to a young patient (18–29 years of age), with a cortical infarct, no history of hypertension or diabetes, no prior stroke or transient ischemic attack (TIA), and is a nonsmoker. On the other hand, older patients with multiple vascular risk factors and an infarct in a deep location will have a lower RoPE score. The "PFO attributable fraction," or the likelihood that a discovered PFO is pathogenically related to the index stroke, ranges from a low of 0% (in the lowest RoPE score strata) to a high of 88% in those with RoPE scores of 9 or 10. Therefore, with the RoPE score, neurologists can be more evidence-based when "presuming" that a stroke was due to paradoxic embolism.

Risk of Paradoxic Embolism Score and Risk of Recurrent Stroke
Risk of stroke recurrence varies with the stroke mechanism. The annual risk of stroke recurrence in patients with index cryptogenic stroke is relatively low, about 1% to 2% per year.[2,14,15] However, this number is reassuring in a misleading way because it does not reflect the accumulated potential of many decades of accrued risk, which is the circumstance for many, often young,

---

Box 4
Risk of paradoxic embolism score calculation
No hypertension (+1)
No diabetes (+1)
No stroke or TIA (+1)
Nonsmoker (+1)
Cortical infarct, on imaging (+1)
Age
18-29 (+5)
30-39 (+4)
40-49 (+3)
50-59 (+2)
60-69 (+1)
$\geq$70 (0)

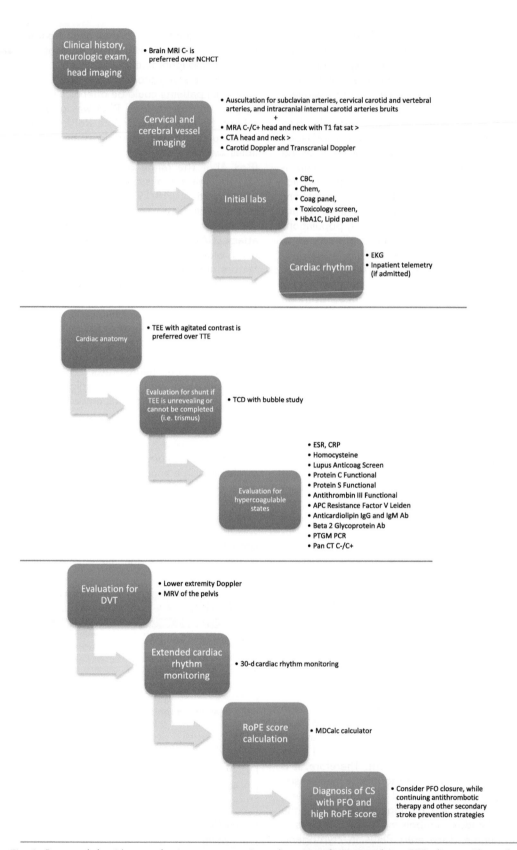

Fig. 1. Proposed algorithm to selecting a cryptogenic stroke patient for transcatheter PFO closure. Ab, antibody; APC, activated protein C; CBC, complete blood count; CRP, C-reactive protein; CS, cryptogenic stroke; CTA,

cryptogenic stroke patients who have many years to live after the index stroke. Among cryptogenic stroke patients with PFO, the risk of recurrence varies by RoPE score. Those with the highest RoPE scores have the lowest risk of recurrence. This may seem counterintuitive, but it reflects simply that cryptogenic stroke is a heterogeneous disorder with many different mechanisms (although all are still formally cryptogenic). It turns out that PFO-related recurrence (high RoPE score strata) is less common than non-PFO-related recurrence (low RoPE score strata). It should *not* be interpreted to mean that PFOs are low risk per se. At an absolute risk of roughly 1% per year, the accumulated risk over a lifetime of a young patient may be very substantial. Therefore, the RoPE score should not be interpreted as an analogue of the CHA_2DS_2-VASc score that predicts stroke risk in patients with atrial fibrillation. A higher RoPE score predicts a *lower* risk of recurrence; the RoPE score does not predict if the PFO is high risk or low risk. The RoPE score should be viewed as a diagnostic tool for PFO relatedness. That is, it is a risk-assessment model to help stratify which cryptogenic stroke patients have an incidental versus a pathogenic PFO.[11,13]

RANDOMIZED EVALUATION OF RECURRENT STROKE COMPARING PATENT FORAMEN OVALE CLOSURE TO ESTABLISHED CURRENT STANDARD OF CARE TREATMENT TRIAL AND TREATMENT SELECTION BASED ON ANATOMIC CHARACTERISTICS

Heterogeneity of treatment effect refers to patient subgroups from within a studied population that benefit differently even though the treatment benefits the group as a whole. The Randomized Evaluation of Recurrent Stroke Comparing PFO Closure to Established Current Standard of Care Treatment (RESPECT) was a multicenter, open-label clinical trial that was designed to demonstrate the superiority of percutaneous PFO closure and medical therapy over medical therapy alone to prevent stroke recurrence in patients with imaging-confirmed cryptogenic stroke and PFO. At a mean follow-up of 5.9 years, PFO closure led to a statistically significant reduction in the risk of recurrent ischemic stroke according to intention-to-treat analysis. One of the assumptions of the RESPECT trial was that patients with PFO-related index events would be likely to have PFO-related recurrences. It became apparent during the course of the trial that approximately one-third of the observed recurrent stroke events were *not* cryptogenic,[15,16] that is, they had a known cause, unrelated to the presence of a PFO. Such strokes could not be prevented with PFO closure. When the extended follow-up data were analyzed in RESPECT after removing the recurrent strokes of known cause (also about one-third of the events), again a significant treatment effect in favor of closure was observed (hazard ratio [HR] 0.38, 95% confidence interval [CI] 0.18–0.79, $P = .007$) as well as when the analysis was limited to patients while they remained less than 60 year old (HR 0.42, 95% CI 0.21–0.83, $P = .010$).

Subgroup analyses of the RESPECT trial suggested heterogeneity of treatment effect, because those patients with large shunts and those with a hypermobile interatrial septum ("atrial septal aneurysm") received particular benefit from PFO closure.[17] Although this argument is compelling, the data from RESPECT should be seen only as hypothesis generating. It should be noted that in the PC (Clinical Trial Comparing Percutaneous Closure of Patent Foramen Ovale [PFO] Using the Amplatzer PFO Occluder with Medical Treatment in Patients with Cryptogenic Embolism) Trial the effect of PFO closure was directed in the opposite direction in the subgroup with hypermobile interatrial septum (ie, more benefit in those *without* atrial septal aneurysms).[18] An individual, patient level, meta-analysis could not identify specific subgroups from the clinical trials who especially benefited, or were harmed, by closure.[19] Therefore, when selecting patients for transcatheter PFO closure, it should be remembered that targeting, or withholding, PFO closure based on echocardiographic parameters is logically compelling, but not yet supported by clinical trial data.

---

computed tomographic angiography; DVT, deep vein thrombosis; EKG, electrocardiogram; ESR, erythrocyte sedimentation rate; HbA1c, hemoglobin A1c; IgG, immunoglobulin G; IgM, immunoglobulin M; MDCalc, MDCalc.com medical calculator; MRI C-, magnetic resonance imaging without contrast; MRI C-/C+, magnetic resonance imaging with and without contrast; MRV, magnetic resonance venography; NCHCT, non-contrast head computed tomography; Pan CT C-/C+, computed tomography with and without contrast from the head to the pubic symphysis; PTGM PCR, prothrombin gene mutation polymerase chain reaction; TCD, transcranial Doppler; TEE, transesophageal echocardiogram; TTE, transthoracic echocardiogram.

PATIENT SELECTION AND US FOOD AND DRUG ADMINISTRATION APPROVAL OF PATENT FORAMEN OVALE CLOSURE FOR CRYPTOGENIC STROKE

Patient selection for PFO closure is evolving, especially since the Amplatzer PFO Occluder (Abbott Vascular, Santa Clara, CA, USA) was approved by the FDA, based upon long-term follow-up of the RESPECT trial, the first PFO closure device approved for stroke prevention in the United States.[20] The RESPECT trial demonstrated a 62% relative risk reduction in recurrent cryptogenic stroke (95% CI 0.18–0.79) compared with medical management in cryptogenic stroke patients with PFO, with a very low risk of safety events.[18,21] In order to achieve rational dispersion (and avoid irrational dispersion) of this technology, proper patient selection is crucial. The FDA label specifically suggests that appropriate patients should be "determined by a neurologist and cardiologist." This wording is an effort to encourage collaboration between the specialties and particularly to recognize that diagnosis of stroke and TIA requires the input of neurologists.

For proper patient selection, the first step is to diagnose a neurologic episode as being due to cerebral, or retinal, ischemia. Next is the obligatory search for potential stroke causes. **Fig. 1** shows a flow chart illustrating one approach to stroke evaluation. If no cause is found and the diagnostic conclusion is "cryptogenic stroke," and a PFO has been discovered, then the RoPE score should be used to estimate the likelihood that the discovered PFO is causally related to the cryptogenic stroke.

SUMMARY

Stroke can be devastating. It is frequent, morbid, and expensive.[1] A stroke with no known mechanism after thorough investigations is called cryptogenic. A cryptogenic stroke with a PFO and a high RoPE score is probably causally related to the PFO. The predictors of stroke recurrence in cryptogenic stroke patients with PFO and high RoPE score include prior stroke, hypermobile septum, and small shunt, but these need further study.[22] The approximate annual recurrence risk in cryptogenic stroke patients with high probability of causal relationship to the PFO is 1%, but that misrepresents what may be a significant accumulated lifetime risk.

The FDA approval of the Amplatzer PFO Occluder for percutaneous transcatheter closure of a PFO, in cryptogenic stroke patients with a high PFO-attributable risk, was granted based on analysis of the longitudinal data from the RESPECT trial. In the intention-to-treat population, there was a 45% relative risk reduction ($P = .046$). The treatment effect was magnified when the outcome was recurrent cryptogenic stroke and when the analysis was limited to patients while they remained less than 60 year old. These analyses support the hypothesis that PFO closure prevents PFO-related recurrent strokes and is associated with fewer recurrences than medical management alone. PFO closure devices are low risk, but *not* no risk. Neurologists and cardiologists must work together to accurately diagnose and select appropriate candidates for PFO closure.

REFERENCES

1. Mozaffarian D, Benjamin EJ, Go AS, et al. Heart Disease and Stroke Statistics—2016 update: a report from the American Heart Association. Circulation 2016;133(4):e38–60.
2. Homma S, Sacco RL. Patent foramen ovale and stroke. Circulation 2005;112:1063–72.
3. Hagen PT, Scholz DG, Edwards WD. Incidence and size of patent foramen ovale during the first 10 decades of life: an autopsy study of 965 normal hearts. Mayo Clin Proc 1984;59:17–20.
4. Meissner I, Khandheria BK, Heit JA, et al. Patent foramen ovale: innocent or guilty? Evidence from a prospective population-based study. J Am Coll Cardiol 2006;47:440–5.
5. Edlow JA, Selim MH. Atypical presentations of acute cerebrovascular syndromes. Lancet Neurol 2011;10(6):550–60.
6. Dupre CM, Libman R, Dupre SI, et al. Stroke chameleons. J Stroke Cerebrovasc Dis 2014;23(2):374–8.
7. Merino JG, Luby M, Benson RT, et al. Predictors of acute stroke mimics in 8187 patients referred to a stroke service. J Stroke Cerebrovasc Dis 2013; 22(8):e397–403.
8. Saver JL. Cryptogenic stroke. N Engl J Med 2016; 374(21):2065–74.
9. O'Donnell M, Kasner SE. Cryptogenic stroke. In: Grotta JC, Albers GW, Broderick JP, et al, editors. STROKE pathophysiology, diagnosis, and management. 6th edition. Amsterdam: Elsevier; 2016. p. 707–15.
10. Hart RG, Diener HC, Coutts SB, et al. Embolic strokes of undetermined source: the case for a new clinical construct. Lancet Neurol 2014;13:429–38.
11. Alsheikh-Ali AA, Thaler DE, Kent DM. Patent foramen ovale in cryptogenic stroke: incidental or pathogenic? Stroke 2009;40(7):2349–55.

12. Thaler DE, Di Angelantonio E, Di Tullio MR, et al. The risk of paradoxical embolism (RoPE) study: initial description of the completed database. Int J Stroke 2013;8(8):612–9.

13. Kent DM, Ruthazer R, Weimar C, et al. An index to identify stroke-related vs incidental patent foramen ovale in cryptogenic stroke. Neurology 2013;81(7): 619–25.

14. Mas JL, Arquizan C, Lamy C, et al. Recurrent cerebrovascular events associated with patent foramen ovale, atrial septal aneurysm, or both. N Engl J Med 2001;345:1740–6.

15. Furlan AJ, Reisman M, Massaro J, et al. Closure or medical therapy for cryptogenic stroke with patent foramen ovale. N Engl J Med 2012;366:991–9.

16. Mattle HP, Mono ML. Closure of a patent foramen ovale with a device does not offer a greater benefit than medical therapy alone for the prevention of recurrent cerebrovascular events. Evid Based Med 2013;18(1):34–5.

17. Caroll JD, Saver JL, Thaler DE, et al. Closure of patent foramen ovale versus medical therapy after cryptogenic stroke. N Engl J Med 2013;368(12):1092–100.

18. Meier B, Kalesan B, Mattle HP, et al. Percutaneous closure of patent foramen ovale in cryptogenic embolism. N Engl J Med 2013;368:1083–91.

19. Kent DM, Dahabreh IJ, Ruthazer R, et al. Device closure of patent foramen ovale after stroke : pooled analysis of completed randomized trials. J Am Coll Cardiol 2016;67(8):907–17.

20. FDA approves new device for prevention of recurrent strokes in certain patients. U.S. Food & Drug Administration Website. 2016. Available at: https://www.fda.gov/NewsEvents/Newsroom/Press Announcements/ucm527096.htm. Accessed March 20, 2016.

21. Thaler D. RESPECT: Final Long-term Outcomes from a Prospective, Randomized Trial of PFO Closure in Patients With Cryptogenic Stroke. Oral presentation at: Transcatheter Cardiovascular Therapeutics Annual Meeting. Washington, DC, November 1, 2016.

22. Thaler DE, Ruthazer R, Weimar C, et al. Recurrent stroke predictors differ in medically treated patients with pathogenic vs other PFOs. Neurology 2014;83(3):221–6.

Identification and Quantification of Patent Foramen Ovale–Mediated Shunts
Echocardiography and Transcranial Doppler

Ahmed N. Mahmoud, MD[a], Islam Y. Elgendy, MD[a],
Nayan Agarwal, MD[a], Jonathan M. Tobis, MD, FACC, MSCAI[b],
Mohammad Khalid Mojadidi, MD[a],*

KEYWORDS

- Patent foramen ovale • Right-to-left shunt • Bubble study • Echocardiography
- Transcranial Doppler

KEY POINTS

- Patent foramen ovale (PFO) is diagnosed using either direct imaging of the interatrial septal defect with echocardiography (transesophageal, transthoracic, or intracardiac echocardiography), or by physiologic quantification of a right-to-left shunt through the PFO using transcranial Doppler.
- Contrast transesophageal echocardiography is considered the standard technique for identifying a PFO and visualizing the atrial septal anatomy, allowing assessment of PFO size and shunt severity, and differentiation between PFO and other right-to-left shunts.
- Transthoracic echocardiography bubble study is the most commonly used method for diagnosing a PFO, being cost-effective and readily available, but with a lower sensitivity.
- Transcranial Doppler is a highly sensitive test that indirectly assesses for the presence of a right-to-left shunt; it is unable to differentiate between cardiac and pulmonary shunts. However, it is the best method to quantitate the severity of right-to-left shunts and is more sensitive than transthoracic and transesophageal echocardiography so is our preferred method of screening for PFO.

INTRODUCTION

The identification and quantification of patent foramen ovale (PFO)–mediated right-to-left shunting is crucial for the management and interventional planning of PFO-associated clinical syndromes. Ultrasonographic assessment of right-to-left shunting, either directly with echocardiography (transthoracic, transesophageal, or intracardiac) or indirectly using transcranial Doppler (TCD), remains the diagnostic approach of choice.[1] Transthoracic echocardiography (TTE) with bubble study is the most commonly used initial imaging modality for the diagnosis

---

Disclosure: Dr J.M. Tobis was a consultant for St. Jude Medical Inc and W.L. Gore Inc. No funding was provided by these companies to write this article. All other authors have no disclosures.
[a] Division of Cardiology, Department of Medicine, University of Florida, 1600 Southwest Archer Road, Gainesville, FL 32608, USA; [b] Division of Cardiology, Department of Medicine, David Geffen School of Medicine at UCLA, 10833 Le Conte Avenue, Factor Building CHS, Room B-976, Los Angeles, CA 90095, USA
* Corresponding author. UF Health, 1600 Southwest Archer Road, North Tower, Room M-430, Gainesville, FL 32608.
E-mail address: mkmojadidi@gmail.com

of PFO.[2–4] Contrast transesophageal echocardiography (TEE) is considered the standard technique for visualizing the atrial septal anatomy, assessment of PFO size and shunt severity, and differentiation between PFO and other right-to-left shunts.[5] TCD is a highly sensitive alternative screening modality to TTE for the diagnosis of PFO-mediated shunting.[6]

This article compares the different available diagnostic modalities and describes the benefits and limitations of the various imaging techniques.

GENERAL PRINCIPLES FOR DETECTION OF RIGHT-TO-LEFT SHUNTING BY ULTRASONOGRAPHY

Ultrasonographic detection of shunting from the right to left atria can be accomplished by TTE, TEE, TCD, or intracardiac echocardiography (ICE). An echocardiographic contrast is injected into the venous circulation while an ultrasonography probe is placed on the patient's chest wall (TTE), in the esophagus (TEE), on the cranium (TCD), or in the right atrium (ICE) to detect Doppler signals generated by the contrast flow. Because normal left atrial pressure is higher than right atrial pressure, a provocation maneuver is necessary to reverse the interatrial pressure gradient and induce a transient right-to-left shunt across a PFO.

Contrast Agents

Agitated saline is the most common contrast agent used for the detection of PFO-mediated right-to-left shunting given its low cost and high efficacy.[7] Agitated saline is prepared by connecting two 10-mL syringes to a 3-way stopcock with one end connected to the patient's intravenous access site. An 18-gauge needle or large bore is preferred to allow a large bolus of contrast to reach the right atrium. One of the 2 syringes is filled with 9 mL of saline and 0.5 to 1 mL of air. The saline and air are then rapidly agitated, by alternating injections between the two syringes at least 5 times, followed by rapid injection of the full bolus into the patient's venous circulation.[7] Addition of a small amount of the patient's blood to the saline before agitation improves the sensitivity of the bubble study; the protein within the plasma permits more microbubbles to remain within a given volume, allowing the contrast to last longer in the patient's circulation. In addition, the air does not coalesce as readily and thus mixing blood reduces the risk of an air embolus and stroke.[8,9] Other contrast agents that have been described in the literature for the detection of right-to-left shunts include gelatin-based solutions, Echovist, hydroxyethylamidon, D-galactose, and Gelifundol.[10–14]

Site of Contrast Injection (Antecubital vs Femoral)

The injection of contrast agent may be performed either through the antecubital vein to the superior vena cava and right atrium or via the femoral vein to the inferior vena cava and right atrium. Each access site has advantages and disadvantages. The femoral route follows the embryologic pathway of oxygenated blood from the placenta directly through the inferior vena cava to the interatrial septum (IAS) and PFO. This direct route may be facilitated by the presence of a residual eustachian valve, and gives femoral access a higher accuracy compared with antecubital access. However, most clinicians do not use femoral injections because of the impracticality of obtaining femoral venous access for a bubble study, except in the cardiac catheterization laboratory. In addition, the use of femoral venous access is discouraged by the Centers for Disease Control and Prevention (CDC), given the higher risk of embolization and infections compared with upper extremity access.[15] Thus, femoral access is usually reserved for either catheter-guided or intraoperative evaluation of right-to-left shunts.[16] Although antecubital access is easier to obtain, it may be associated with lower diagnostic accuracy than femoral access, because the contrast agent could flow from the superior vena cava to the right atrium and directly through the tricuspid valve without reaching the IAS, especially with the presence of a persistent eustachian valve.[7]

Provocation Maneuvers

Unlike atrial septal defects (ASDs), right-to-left PFO shunts are usually transient and occur when right-sided cardiac pressure increases, resulting in a reversal in interatrial pressure gradient (eg, during coughing or after release of the Valsalva maneuver). Thus, provocation maneuvers are necessary during ultrasonographic evaluation of a PFO to reveal this transient shunt that would otherwise remain undetected. A commonly used provocation maneuver is asking the patient to perform a Valsalva maneuver either during or immediately after injection of the contrast agent. However, patients are often unable to perform a Valsalva maneuver during a TEE in the setting of conscious sedation and with a probe in the esophagus. In these situations, other provocation maneuvers can be performed, such as maintaining gentle abdominal pressure for 10 to 20 seconds and then releasing it during or immediately after contrast injection. The release of the Valsalva maneuver permits the sudden return of venous blood to the right atrium with right atrial pressure transiently exceeding left atrial pressure.[17]

Criteria for Diagnosis of Intracardiac Right-to-Left Shunts

The diagnosis of intracardiac right-to-left shunting is confirmed when microbubbles are seen in either the left atrium or ventricle (TTE and TEE) or the middle cerebral arteries (TCD) after injection of contrast and a provocation maneuver. The exact number of microbubbles that correspond with a positive test is not well defined and varies from one institution to another; a positive TTE or TEE is considered if at least 1 to 5 microbubbles are visualized after 3 to 5 cardiac cycles after complete opacification of the right atrium following contrast injection and provocation.[18–21] Despite some interinstitutional variability, most clinicians accept that a positive intracardiac right-to-left shunt comprises the passage of 1 or more microbubbles into the left atrium within 3 cardiac cycles. Microbubbles passing to the left cardiac chambers after 3 cardiac cycles may indicate the presence of an intrapulmonary rather than an intracardiac shunt. The TCD criteria for diagnosis of intracardiac shunt are better defined, more sensitive, and are discussed in detail later.

DIAGNOSIS OF RIGHT-TO-LEFT SHUNT BY TRANSTHORACIC ECHOCARDIOGRAPHY

TTE is the most common initial screening modality for the detection of right-to-left shunts primarily because it is most readily available, but it has the poorest sensitivity.[2,3,22] Given the posterior position of both atria, direct visualization of interatrial shunts by color Doppler provides a lower yield; agitated saline bubble study is thus the technique of choice.[23–25]

Transthoracic Echocardiography Protocol for Detecting Right-to-Left Shunt

1. The TTE probe is placed either at the apical 4-chamber or subxiphoid 4-chamber views.
2. The agitated saline contrast agent is then injected into the patient's antecubital vein, while acquiring a prolonged image by TTE.
3. After the first study is performed at rest, a second study is obtained during a Valsalva maneuver. The test is considered positive if microbubbles are visualized in the left

atrium or ventricle within 3 to 5 cardiac cycles after complete opacification of the right atrium (**Fig. 1**).

Diagnostic Accuracy of Transthoracic Echocardiography for Detection of Intracardiac Right-to-Left Shunt

Multiple factors affect the sensitivity and specificity of TTE bubble studies. In general, TTE bubble study is characterized by a high specificity (except if a pulmonary arteriovenous malformation is present), making it an acceptable rule-in test.[4,26] Although the sensitivity of fundamental TTE is much lower than that of TEE for the detection of right-to-left shunt, modern echocardiography uses second harmonic imaging, which has improved the sensitivity of the TTE bubble study.[26]

In a meta-analysis of 13 prospective studies including 1436 patients, the overall weighted sensitivity of fundamental TTE for the detection of intracardiac right-to-left shunts was 46.4% (95% confidence interval [CI], 41.1%–51.8%) and specificity was 99.2% (95% CI, 98.4%–99.7%) compared with TEE as the reference. The sensitivity and specificity were not affected by different contrast agents, different cutoffs for the minimum number of bubbles that determine a positive test, or different cutoffs for the number of cardiac cycles that determine a positive test.[4] In contrast, a meta-analysis including 15 prospective studies determined that TTE with harmonic imaging has a sensitivity of 90.5% (95% CI, 88.1%–92.6%) and specificity of 92.6% (95% CI, 91.0%–94.0%), compared

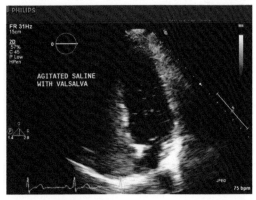

Fig. 1. Positive transthoracic echocardiogram (apical 4-chamber view) bubble study in a 33-year old patient with severe migraine with visual aura. (*From* Mojadidi MK, Gevorgyan R, Tobis JM. A comparison of methods to detect and quantitate PFO: TCD, TTE, ICE and TEE. In: Amin Z, Tobis JM, Sievert H, et al, editors. Patent foramen ovale. London: Springer; 2015. p. 55–65; with permission.)

with TEE as the reference. A cutoff of 1 or more microbubbles (instead of ≥5), within 3 cardiac cycles (instead of 5), resulted in a higher specificity of TTE harmonic imaging without compromising sensitivity. In addition, the mixture of a patient's blood to agitated saline increases the sensitivity of TTE harmonic imaging without compromising specificity.[26] Table 1 summarizes the diagnostic accuracy of TTE (with and without harmonic imaging) for the detection of intracardiac right-to-left shunt compared with TEE as the reference. However, all of these studies are flawed because the true comparison for the diagnosis of a PFO should be a right heart catheterization with documentation of passage of a guidewire across the atrial septum. However, few studies have been performed with right heart catheterization as the gold standard.

Advantages and Disadvantages of Transthoracic Echocardiography for Detection of Intracardiac Right-to-Left Shunt

Advantages of TTE bubble study include its noninvasive nature, easy availability, lower cost (compared with TEE), and high specificity. However, TTE is limited by a lower sensitivity, low resolution, and poor visualization of the IAS. Table 2 shows the advantages and disadvantages of TTE for detection of intracardiac right-to-left shunt.

Although TTE bubble study is the most common screening modality for the detection of PFO-mediated right-to-left shunting, its lower sensitivity, often poor acoustic windows, and poorly visualized IAS make it a less than ideal screening test. PFOs are often missed if

clinicians rely on TTE alone; alternative screening such as TCD or use of TTE with TEE is often necessary to make a definitive diagnosis.

PATENT FORAMEN OVALE IMAGING BY TRANSESOPHAGEAL ECHOCARDIOGRAPHY

TEE is considered by many clinicians to be the standard for diagnosing a PFO.[1,27] TEE provides anatomic details of the IAS and can differentiate a PFO from an ASD but may still incorrectly diagnose pulmonary shunts.[1] Moreover, TEE can more accurately detect the presence of an atrial septal aneurysm compared with TTE. The presence of a PFO with an atrial septal aneurysm has been linked to a higher risk of cryptogenic stroke.[28,29] In patients with stroke, TEE can detect other sources of embolism (left ventricular thrombus, aortic plaque burden, and left atrial appendage clot) that may otherwise be missed by TTE.

Transesophageal Echocardiography Protocol for Detecting a Patent Foramen Ovale

1. The IAS is first visualized in multiple views (ie, bicaval, 4 chamber, short and long axis) using multiplane angles for accurate determination of the IAS anatomy and ruling out other causes of stroke or hypoxemia.
2. Both the 4 chamber and bicaval views can be used for direct visualization of the PFO.
3. Agitated saline contrast is injected in a similar fashion as described with TTE. Because it is often difficult for the patient to perform an adequate Valsalva maneuver with sedation and a probe in the esophagus, transient external abdominal pressure can be applied over the liver for 10 to 20 seconds, which is then released during or immediately after injecting contrast to increase intrathoracic and right atrial pressure.
4. The test is considered positive if at least 1 microbubble is seen in the left atrium with evidence of transient opening of the PFO canal during the first 3 cardiac cycles, after injection of agitated saline and complete opacification of the right atrium (Fig. 2). The international consensus for TEE grading is often used to quantify the size of shunts[17] (Table 3).

Diagnostic Accuracy of Transesophageal Echocardiography for Detection of Patent Foramen Ovale

Although TEE bubble study is considered the gold standard noninvasive modality for detecting a PFO, one study comparing TEE with PFO

Table 1
Diagnostic accuracies of transthoracic echocardiography, transcranial Doppler, and transesophageal echocardiography bubble studies for the detection of intracardiac right-to-left shunt

	Sensitivity (%)	Specificity (%)	LR+	LR−
TTE-F[4]	46	99	20.85	0.57
TTE-HI[26]	91	93	13.52	0.13
TCD[6]	97	93	13.51	0.04
TEE[5]	89	91	5.93	0.22

TTE-F, TTE-HI, and TCD compared with TEE as the reference standard. TEE compared with PFO confirmation by cardiac catheterization, surgery, and/or autopsy as the reference standard.

Abbreviations: TTE-F, fundamental TTE; TTE-HI, TTE with harmonic imaging; LR+, positive likelihood ratio; LR−, negative likelihood ratio.

Table 2
Advantages and disadvantages of transthoracic echocardiography, transcranial Doppler, and transesophageal echocardiography for the diagnosis of patent foramen ovale

	Advantages	Disadvantages
TTE	• Readily available • Cost-effective • Excellent safety • Easy to perform	• Low resolution • Less sensitive than TCD • Images may be limited by patient's body habitus and poor echocardiographic windows • Often difficult to differentiate between PFO, ASD, and pulmonary shunts
TCD	• Highly sensitive • Cost-effective • Excellent safety • Easy to perform	• Positive test based on an arbitrary cutoff • Inability to differentiate between PFO, ASD, and pulmonary shunts (ie, lower specificity) • Inability to visualize atrial septum
TEE	• Highly accurate imaging modality • Can visualize atrial septal anatomy • Accurate assessment of PFO size • Accurate assessment of shunt severity • Differentiates PFO from ASD and pulmonary shunts • Useful for closure planning • In addition to diagnosing PFO, can detect other sources of embolism	• Semi-invasive procedure • Need for sedation • Difficulty performing Valsalva with a probe in the esophagus • Carries a risk of complications • May not be used in patients with esophageal stricture, cancer, or varices • Difficulty in uncooperative patients with swallowing dysfunction

confirmation by autopsy found TEE to have a sensitivity of 89%.[30] Studies comparing TEE with PFO confirmation during cardiac catheterization or intraoperative detection similarly found that 10% of PFOs are missed by TEE.[31–34] In a meta-analysis of 4 prospective studies comparing TEE with PFO confirmation by surgery, right heart catheterization, and/or autopsy, TEE had a weighted sensitivity of 89.2% (95% CI, 81.1–94.7) and specificity of 91.4% (95% CI, 82.3%–96.8%), indicating that approximately 10% of PFOs are either missed or misdiagnosed if the clinician relies on TEE alone.[5] This finding

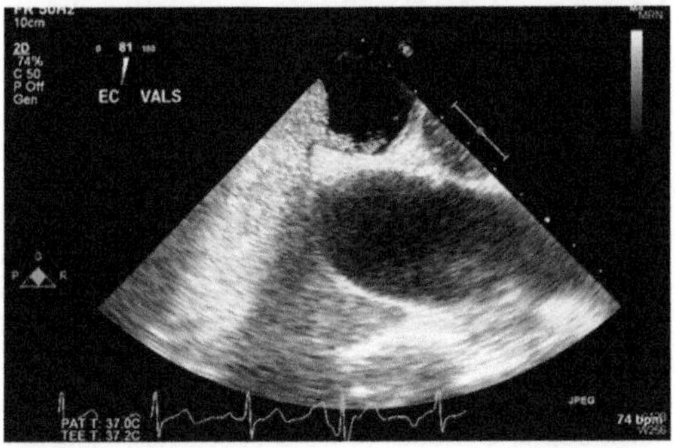

may be explained by the difficulty of performing a Valsalva maneuver with a TEE probe in the patient's esophagus, at times poor patient compliance, different patient anatomies, and operator experience.

Advantages and Disadvantages of Transesophageal Echocardiography

Advantages of TEE include accurate description of the IAS anatomy, ability to detect an aneurysmal atrial septum, differentiating a PFO from an ASD, PFO sizing, and functional assessment of shunt severity by color flow Doppler or agitated saline bubble study. However, TEE is an uncomfortable procedure requiring conscious sedation. TEE also carries a risk of bleeding and perforation, particularly in patients with known esophageal disorders such as varices, strictures, and achalasia.[34] Table 2 summarizes the advantages and disadvantages of TEE for PFO imaging.

Fig. 2. Transesophageal echocardiogram with positive bubble study through a PFO. (*From* Mojadidi MK, Gevorgyan R, Tobis JM. A comparison of methods to detect and quantitate PFO: TCD, TTE, ICE and TEE. In: Amin Z, Tobis JM, Sievert H, et al, editors. Patent foramen ovale. London: Springer; 2015. p. 55–65; with permission.)

Table 3
International consensus for transthoracic echocardiography grading

Grade	mB
Grade 0	None
Grade 1	1–10
Grade 2	10–20
Grade 3	>20; curtain appearance of mB

Abbreviation: Mb, microbubbles.

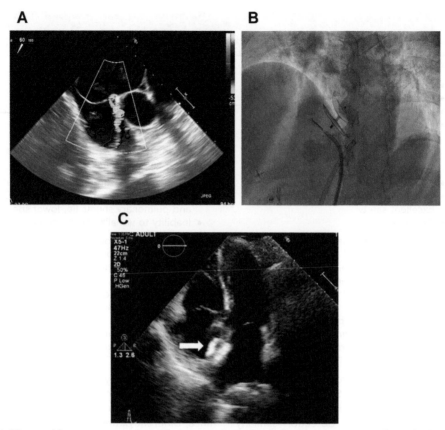

Fig. 3. A 38-year-old woman presenting with cryptogenic stroke. Color Doppler transesophageal echocardiography images revealed a significant left-to-right shunt through a PFO (*A*). Bubble study was positive for transient right-to-left shunting. The patient underwent successful percutaneous PFO closure with an Amplatzer Multifenestrated (Cribiform) Septal Occluder (St Jude Medical, St. Paul, MN) seen on fluoroscopy (*B*) and transthoracic echocardiography (*arrow in C*).

In summary, TEE offers an acceptable diagnostic accuracy compared with autopsy, cardiac catheterization, and/or surgical detection of PFO. The main advantage of TEE is the anatomic determination of PFO structure and ruling out other causes of right-to-left shunting. Thus, TEE is an excellent confirmatory tool for identification and evaluation of PFO-mediated shunting, after an initial noninvasive screening modality (Figs. 3 and 4). However, clinicians should be aware that the diagnosis of a PFO by TEE alone may be misleading. If the clinical scenario justifies a higher level of certainty, a right heart catheterization may be necessary to determine an accurate diagnosis.

DIAGNOSIS OF INTRACARDIAC RIGHT-TO-LEFT SHUNT BY TRANSCRANIAL DOPPLER

TCD bubble study is an alternative imaging modality for indirectly detecting a PFO by assessing for the presence of right-to-left shunting. It

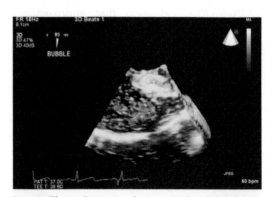

Fig. 4. Three-dimensional transesophageal echocardiographic image after placement of a 25-mm Gore Helex Septal Occluder (Gore & Associates, Flagstaff, AZ). During agitated saline bubble study, bubbles are visualized in the right atrium, but not on the left atrial side. (*From* Mojadidi MK, Gevorgyan R, Tobis JM. A comparison of methods to detect and quantitate PFO: TCD, TTE, ICE and TEE. In: Amin Z, Tobis JM, Sievert H, et al, editors. Patent foramen ovale. London: Springer; 2015. p. 55–65; with permission.)

Table 4	
Spencer Logarithmic Scale for transcranial Doppler grading	
Grade	**mB**
Grade 0	0
Grade 1	1–10
Grade 2	11–30
Grade 3	31–100
Grade 4	101–300
Grade 5	>300

allows functional assessment of the shunt through insonation of the middle cerebral arteries after venous injection of agitated saline and release of the Valsalva maneuver. The degree of shunting with TCD can be quantified by using the Spencer logarithmic scale. The Spencer scale scores the severity of shunts using 5 grades (0–5) with 0 being absence of a shunt and 5 being consistent with a large shunt (Table 4). Based on a comparative study with right heart catheterization, a TCD is considered positive if the score is grade 3 or higher on the Spencer scale.[31] Lower grades usually correlate to small, clinically insignificant pulmonary shunts or pinhole septal defects. Modern TCDs are fitted with power M-mode software, which allows better microbubble signal detection, and therefore a more accurate quantification of right-to-left shunting. Studies comparing power M-mode TCD with older TCD models show that power M-mode TCD has a higher sensitivity and accuracy.[31]

Transcranial Doppler Protocol for Detecting Intracardiac Right-to-Left Shunt

1. The TCD ultrasonography probe is placed in an acoustic window (eg, transtemporal, transorbital, or suboccipital window) (Fig. 5).

2. Agitated saline is injected into the antecubital vein and the patient is asked to perform a Valsalva maneuver.

3. The circulation of microbubbles in the insonated vessel is visualized by M-mode Doppler and the grade of right-to-left shunt is quantified over 1 minute using the Spencer logarithmic scale (Fig. 6).

Diagnostic Accuracy of Transcranial Doppler for Detecting Intracardiac Right-to-Left Shunts

TCD is a highly sensitive imaging modality for detection of intracardiac right-to-left shunts. In a study comparing TCD and TEE bubble studies versus PFO probing during right heart catheterization, TCD was more sensitive than TEE.[31] In a large meta-analysis of 27 prospective studies including 1968 patients, TCD bubble study had a sensitivity of 97% (95% CI, 94%–98%) and specificity of 93% (95% CI, 86%–97%) for the detection of intracardiac right-to-left shunts compared with TEE as the reference.[6]

Advantages and Disadvantages of Transcranial Doppler for Detection of Intracardiac Right-to-Left Shunt

Besides its high sensitivity, TCD provides useful information on the size of the shunt using the Spencer scale. In addition, TCD is easily tolerated, cost-effective, and safe. The indirect functional assessment for a shunt without anatomic imaging of the atrial septum limits TCD in differentiating between a PFO, ASD, and pulmonary shunts; this largely explains the lower specificity of TCD. Table 2 summarizes the advantages and disadvantages of TCD for the detection of intracardiac right-to-left shunts.

In summary, TCD is a highly sensitive diagnostic modality that is cost-effective and easy to perform. These qualities make TCD an

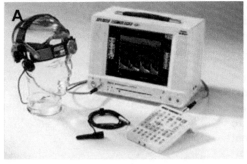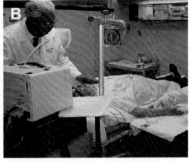

Fig. 5. (A) TCD machine and setup. (B) Dr Spencer demonstrates the technique for TCD that he developed. The patient is supine with a headband on and an intravenous line in the right antecubital fossa. The power M-mode equipment shows the headband, ultrasonography transducers, and the arterial waveform on Doppler. (*Courtesy of* Spencer Technologies, Redmond, WA; with permission.)

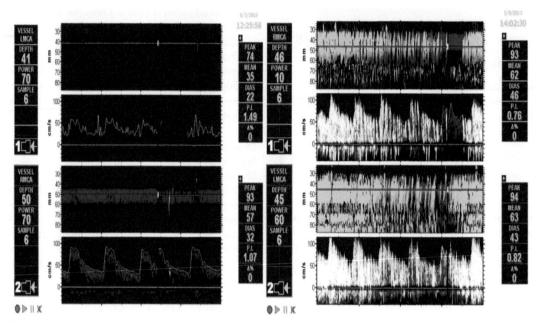

Fig. 6. TCD grading with microembolic signals that measure degree of right-to-left shunting ranging from grade 1 (*left*) to grade 5 (*right*).

excellent initial screening modality for the detection of PFO. A positive test with TCD, although accurate in detecting a right-to-left shunt, carries the possibility of being a false-positive for the presence of a PFO either from an ASD or intrapulmonary shunt. TCD is an indirect functional test that does not visualize the IAS and thus a confirmatory test either with TEE or ICE (during percutaneous PFO closure) should be performed following a positive TCD.

OTHER DIAGNOSTIC MODALITIES FOR IDENTIFICATION AND QUANTIFICATION OF A PATENT FORAMEN OVALE

ICE and cardiac MRI are other imaging options that are used for both anatomic visualization of the IAS and evaluation of right-to-left shunting. ICE has emerged as an invasive imaging modality that is primarily used during transcatheter PFO closure.[35] A PFO is visualized with ICE in a horizontal view of the septum posterior to the aortic bulge (Fig. 7).[36] Advantages of ICE include highly detailed visualization of the IAS, low procedure cost, no need for general anesthesia, and the ability of the interventionist to control the ICE probe without the requirement of another specialist during the procedure.[1] ICE is also useful for the immediate detection of residual shunting after percutaneous PFO closure (Fig. 8). Disadvantages include the need for a second venous access, increasing

the risk of vascular access–related complications. In a study comparing ICE with TEE, ICE had a similar preclosure right-to-left shunt detection rate. However, the detection rate was much lower following device closure, which could be attributed to the monoplane nature of ICE or the presence of a device between the ICE probe and contrast microbubbles, resulting in a lower image yield.[37]

Cardiac MRI is less frequently used as an imaging modality for the detection of PFO, given the low sensitivity of MRI compared with TEE.

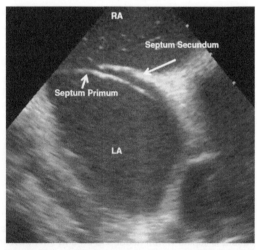

Fig. 7. Patent foramen ovale shown on ICE. LA, left atrium; RA, right atrium.

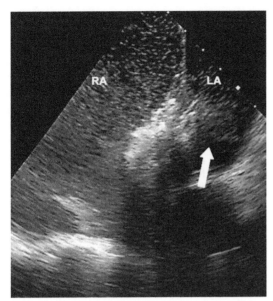

Fig. 8. Gore Helex Septal Occluder with moderate residual shunting (*arrow*) through the device on ICE.

The low sensitivity of MRI may be explained by a lack of continuous and prolonged images that are required given the transient nature of right-to-left shunting across a PFO.[38,39]

SUMMARY AND RECOMMENDATIONS

TCD bubble study has the highest sensitivity for the detection of PFO-mediated right-to-left shunt, making it the initial screening modality of choice. In centers where TCD is unavailable, TTE with harmonic imaging can be used for initial screening, keeping in mind that a significant fraction of PFOs are missed with TTE. A subsequent TEE bubble study will provide additional information on IAS anatomy before transcutaneous or surgical closure. If TEE is not feasible because of contraindications or patient intolerance, ICE can be used during percutaneous PFO closure. Cardiac MRI should not be routinely used for the detection of PFO given its low sensitivity and high cost compared with other available imaging modalities.

REFERENCES

1. Silvestry FE, Cohen MS, Armsby LB, et al, American Society of Echocardiography, Society for Cardiac Angiography and Interventions. Guidelines for the echocardiographic assessment of atrial septal defect and patent foramen ovale: from the American Society of Echocardiography and Society for Cardiac Angiography and Interventions. J Am Soc Echocardiogr 2015;28:910–58.
2. Belkin RN, Pollack BD, Ruggiero ML, et al. Comparison of transesophageal and transthoracic echocardiography with contrast and color flow Doppler in the detection of patent foramen ovale. Am Heart J 1994;128:520–5.
3. Zito C, Dattilo G, Oreto G, et al. Patent foramen ovale: comparison among diagnostic strategies in cryptogenic stroke and migraine. Echocardiography 2009;26:495–503.
4. Mojadidi MK, Winoker JS, Roberts SC, et al. Accuracy of conventional transthoracic echocardiography for the diagnosis of intracardiac right-to-left shunt: a meta-analysis of prospective studies. Echocardiography 2014;31:1036–48.
5. Mojadidi MK, Bogush N, Caceres JD, et al. Diagnostic accuracy of transesophageal echocardiogram for the detection of patent foramen ovale: a meta-analysis. Echocardiography 2014;31:752–8.
6. Mojadidi MK, Roberts SC, Winoker JS, et al. Accuracy of transcranial Doppler for the diagnosis of intracardiac right-to-left shunt: a bivariate meta-analysis of prospective studies. JACC Cardiovasc Imaging 2014;7:236–50.
7. Mojadidi MK, Gevorgyan R, Tobis JM. A comparison of methods to detect and quantitate PFO: TCD, TTE, ICE and TEE. In: Amin Z, Tobis JM, Sievert H, et al, editors. Patent foramen ovale. London: Springer; 2015. p. 55–65.
8. Fan S, Nagai T, Luo H, et al. Superiority of the combination of blood and agitated saline for routine contrast enhancement. J Am Soc Echocardiogr 1999;12:94–8.
9. Mojadidi MK, Zhang L, Chugh Y, et al. Transcranial Doppler: does addition of blood to agitated saline affect sensitivity for detecting cardiac right-to-left shunt? Echocardiography 2016;33(8):1219–27.
10. Hausmann D, Mügge A, Becht I, et al. Diagnosis of patent foramen ovale by transesophageal echocardiography and association with cerebral and peripheral embolic events. Am J Cardiol 1992;70:668–72.
11. Buttignoni SC, Khorsand A, Mundigler G, et al. Agitated saline versus polygelatine for the echocardiographic assessment of patent foramen ovale. J Am Soc Echocardiogr 2004;17:1059–65.
12. Kühl HP, Hoffmann R, Merx MW, et al. Transthoracic echocardiography using second harmonic imaging: diagnostic alternative to transesophageal echocardiography for the detection of atrial right to left shunt in patients with cerebral embolic events. J Am Coll Cardiol 1999;34:1823–30.
13. Lefèvre J, Lafitte S, Reant P, et al. Optimization of patent foramen ovale detection by contrast transthoracic echocardiography using second harmonic imaging. Arch Cardiovasc Dis 2008;101:213–9.

14. Stendel R, Gramm HJ, Schröder K, et al. Transcranial Doppler ultrasonography as a screening technique for detection of a patent foramen ovale before surgery in the sitting position. Anesthesiology 2000;93:971–5.

15. O'Grady NP, Alexander M, Dellinger EP, et al. Guidelines for the prevention of intravascular catheter-related infections. Infect Control Hosp Epidemiol 2002;23:759–69.

16. Gevorgyan R, Perlowski A, Shenoda M, et al. Sensitivity of brachial versus femoral vein injection of agitated saline to detect right-to-left shunts with transcranial Doppler. Catheter Cardiovasc Interv 2014;84:992–6.

17. Lao AY, Sharma VK, Tsivgoulis G, et al. Detection of right-to-left shunts: comparison between the International Consensus and Spencer Logarithmic Scale criteria. J Neuroimaging 2008;18:402–6.

18. Nemec JJ, Marwick TH, Lorig RJ, et al. Comparison of transcranial Doppler ultrasound and transesophageal contrast echocardiography in the detection of interatrial right-to-left shunts. Am J Cardiol 1991;68:1498–502.

19. Thanigaraj S, Valika A, Zajarias A, et al. Comparison of transthoracic versus transesophageal echocardiography for detection of right-to-left atrial shunting using agitated saline contrast. Am J Cardiol 2005; 96:1007–10.

20. Clarke NR, Timperley J, Kelion AD, et al. Transthoracic echocardiography using second harmonic imaging with Valsalva manoeuvre for the detection of right to left shunts. Eur J Echocardiogr 2004;5: 176–81.

21. Daniëls C, Weytjens C, Cosyns B, et al. Second harmonic transthoracic echocardiography: the new reference screening method for the detection of patent foramen ovale. Eur J Echocardiogr 2004;5:449–52.

22. Souteyrand G, Motreff P, Lusson JR, et al. Comparison of transthoracic echocardiography using second harmonic imaging, transcranial Doppler and transesophageal echocardiography for the detection of patent foramen ovale in stroke patients. Eur J Echocardiogr 2006;7:147–54.

23. Attaran RR, Ata I, Kudithipudi V, et al. Protocol for optimal detection and exclusion of a patent foramen ovale using transthoracic echocardiography with agitated saline microbubbles. Echocardiography 2006;23:616–22.

24. Johansson MC, Helgason H, Dellborg M, et al. Sensitivity for detection of patent foramen ovale increased with increasing number of contrast injections: a descriptive study with contrast transesophageal echocardiography. J Am Soc Echocardiogr 2008;21:419–24.

25. Marriott K, Manins V, Forshaw A, et al. Detection of right-to-left atrial communication using agitated saline contrast imaging: experience with 1162 patients and recommendations for echocardiography. J Am Soc Echocardiogr 2013;26:96–102.

26. Mojadidi MK, Winoker JS, Roberts SC, et al. Two-dimensional echocardiography using second harmonic imaging for the diagnosis of intracardiac right-to-left shunt: a meta-analysis of prospective studies. Int J Cardiovasc Imaging 2014;30:911–23.

27. Seiler C. How should we assess patent foramen ovale? Heart 2004;90:1245–7.

28. Overell JR, Bone I, Lees KR. Interatrial septal abnormalities and stroke: a meta-analysis of case-control studies. Neurology 2000;55:1172–9.

29. Wahl A, Krumsdorf U, Meier B, et al. Transcatheter treatment of atrial septal aneurysm associated with patent foramen ovale for prevention of recurrent paradoxical embolism in high-risk patients. J Am Coll Cardiol 2005;45:377–80.

30. Schneider B, Zienkiewicz T, Jansen V, et al. Diagnosis of patent foramen ovale by transesophageal echocardiography and correlation with autopsy findings. Am J Cardiol 1996;77:1202–9.

31. Spencer MP, Moehring MA, Jesurum J, et al. Power m-mode transcranial Doppler for diagnosis of patent foramen ovale and assessing transcatheter closure. J Neuroimaging 2004;14:342–9.

32. Augoustides JG, Weiss SJ, Weiner J, et al. Diagnosis of patent foramen ovale with multiplane transesophageal echocardiography in adult cardiac surgical patients. J Cardiothorac Vasc Anesth 2004;18:725–30.

33. Chen WJ, Kuan P, Lien WP, et al. Detection of patent foramen ovale by contrast transesophageal echocardiography. Chest 1992;101:1515–20.

34. Mathur SK, Singh P. Transoesophageal echocardiography related complications. Indian J Anaesth 2009;53:567–74.

35. Bartel T, Müller S. Device closure of interatrial communications: peri-interventional echocardiographic assessment. Eur Heart J Cardiovasc Imaging 2013; 14:618–24.

36. Hijazi ZM, Shivkumar K, Sahn DJ. Intracardiac echocardiography during interventional and electrophysiological cardiac catheterization. Circulation 2009;119:587–96.

37. Johansson MC, Eriksson P, Guron CW, et al. Pitfalls in diagnosing PFO: characteristics of false-negative contrast injections during transesophageal echocardiography in patients with patent foramen ovales. J Am Soc Echocardiogr 2010;23:1136–42.

38. Hamilton-Craig C, Sestito A, Natale L, et al. Contrast transoesophageal echocardiography remains superior to contrast-enhanced cardiac magnetic resonance imaging for the diagnosis of patent foramen ovale. Eur J Echocardiogr 2011;12:222–7.

39. Mojadidi MK, Mahmoud AN, Elgendy IY, et al. Transesophageal echocardiography for the detection of patent foramen ovale. J Am Soc Echocardiogr 2017. http://dx.doi.org/10.1016/j.echo.2017.05.006.

Imaging Assessment of the Interatrial Septum for Transcatheter Atrial Septal Defect and Patent Foramen Ovale Closure

Mary Z. Bechis, MD, David S. Rubenson, MD, Matthew J. Price, MD*

KEYWORDS

- Atrial septal defect • Patent foramen ovale • Transesophageal echocardiography
- Intracardiac echocardiography • Intraprocedural echocardiography • Interatrial septum

---

KEY POINTS

- The patent foramen ovale is a normal fetal interatrial connection that persists into adulthood with a septal flap that intermittently opens to enable a right-to-left shunt.
- Atrial septal defects (ASDs) are deficiencies of the interatrial septum (IAS) with the secundum type being the most common and amenable to percutaneous device closure.
- The dimensions and features of the ASD and the presence or absence of its 5 surrounding rims (superior vena cava, retroaortic, atrioventricular valve, inferior vena cava, and posterior free wall) are essential to determine anatomic suitability and device selection for percutaneous closure.
- Intraprocedural echocardiographic guidance assesses for successful device deployment and monitors for procedural complications, the most common of which is cardiac perforation resulting in pericardial effusion and possible tamponade.
- A deficient retroaortic rim and ASDs high within the IAS with deficient superior rims are most commonly identified in cases of device erosions, and warrant special consideration for procedural planning and assessment of the final device position.

INTRODUCTION

Transcatheter closure of atrial septal defects (ASDs) and patent foramen ovale (PFO) has become increasingly common in the last decade with advances in device and imaging technology. The percutaneous approach is now the preferred method of closure when anatomically suitable. Two-dimensional (2D) and 3-dimensional (3D) echocardiography are used to determine this anatomic suitability by characterizing the interatrial defect and its surrounding structures, and are also critical for intraprocedural guidance and postprocedure follow-up. This article provides an overview of interatrial anatomy as it pertains to interventional considerations and discusses the 3 echocardiographic modalities used for periprocedural and intraprocedural imaging of the interatrial septum (IAS): transthoracic echocardiography (TTE), transesophageal echocardiography (TEE), and intracardiac echocardiography (ICE).

Disclosure Statement: No relevant disclosures (M.Z. Bechis and D.S. Rubenson). Honoraria for consulting and proctor services from St. Jude Medical and honoraria from consulting from W.L. Gore (M.J. Price).
Division of Cardiovascular Diseases, Scripps Clinic, 9898 Genesee Avenue, La Jolla, CA 92037, USA
* Corresponding author. 9898 Genesee Avenue, AMP-200, La Jolla, CA 92037.
E-mail address: price.matthew@scrippshealth.org

ANATOMY OF THE INTERATRIAL SEPTUM AND COMMON DEFECTS

Early in embryonic life, the IAS is formed as the septum primum migrates from the atrial roof toward the endocardial cushions that create the atrioventricular (AV) junction. Fenestrations form and coalesce on the superior aspect of the septum primum to form the ostium secundum that maintains the interatrial communication and becomes the foramen ovale for the remainder of fetal life. Next, the septum secundum develops from infolding of the atrial roof as an outer rim that overlaps and eventually fuses with the septum primum except for the inferior aspect. This thin nonoverlapping portion of the septum, composed only of the septum primum, is the fossa ovalis (Fig. 1).

Patent Foramen Ovale

The foramen ovale is a potential space formed by a flap of the septum primum over the septum secundum in the anterior-superior portion of the IAS. This normal fetal configuration allows oxygenated blood from the inferior vena cava (IVC) to bypass the immature fetal pulmonary system and cross into the systemic left heart circulation. After birth, the pressure differential between the left atrium (LA) and right atrium (RA) closes the septum primum flap over the septum secundum, which usually fuses within the first year of life. However, a PFO persists in approximately 25% of the adult population.[1–3] The septal flap usually remains closed against the septum secundum by higher left atrial pressures but may transiently open to right-to-left shunt with respiration, Valsalva, or any other maneuver

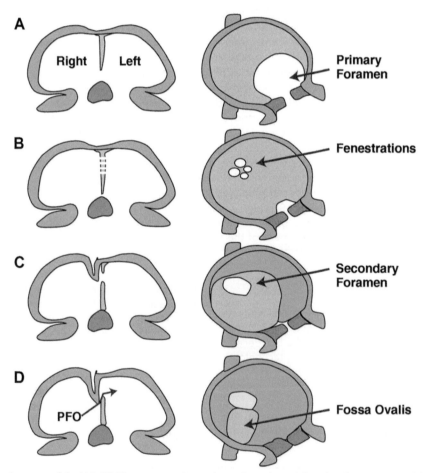

Fig. 1. Development of the IAS. (A) The septum primum forms from the atrial roof and grows toward the endocardial cushions. (B) Fenestrations develop to form the ostium secundum followed by the infolding of the atrial roof to become the rim of septum secundum. (C) The septum primum and septum secundum fuse except for the inferior aspect where the septum primum becomes the fossa ovalis. (D) The foramen ovale is a fetal connection at the anterior-superior aspect of the fossa ovalis. (From Rana BS, Thomas MR, Calvert PA, et al. Echocardiographic evaluation of patent foramen ovale before device closure. JACC Cardiovasc Imaging 2010;3(7):752; with permission from Elsevier.)

that increases venous return and elevates the right atrial pressure. A stretched PFO exhibits intermittent or continuous left-to-right flow due to atrial enlargement and elevated left atrial pressures (Fig. 2).

For considerations of percutaneous closure, PFOs are morphologically categorized into simple versus complex (Fig. 3). Characteristics that define a complex PFO include atrial septal aneurysms (ASAs), long tunnel lengths, multiple fenestrations or other defects of the fossa ovalis, a thickened septum secundum, or prominent Eustachian ridge. These features pose structural challenges that must be considered in device selection and carefully assessed during device deployment to ensure adequate seal.

ASA is redundant septal primum tissue with excessive mobility of the fossa ovalis. ASA is defined as excursion of greater than 10 mm into either the LA or RA or a total excursion of 15 mm in septal motion. The prevalence of ASA in the general population is approximately 2% to 3%.[4] ASA increases the likelihood of the presence of PFO and, in some studies, is associated with higher risk of thromboembolic stroke. Patients with ASA are also more likely to have larger PFOs or complex PFOs with multiple fenestrations. In addition to the need to cover larger and potentially multifenestrated PFOs, the aneurysmal septal tissue itself often requires larger device sizes to stabilize the surrounding rims to ensure complete occlusion of the shunt after device placement.

PFOs with rigid tunnels of length greater than 10 mm may pose difficulty for successful device closure because the device may not align correctly with the IAS after deployment and release. A wide opening on either end of the tunnel risks inadequate seal, or even embolization, if not accounted for by the placement of a larger device size. PFOs with multiple fenestrations or hybrid defects that are associated with ASDs may require larger or multiple devices to fully seal. A prominent septum secundum or lipomatous hypertrophy of the IAS may hinder the ability of the device to grab the septum in a stable fashion, leading to device shifting, residual leak, and possible embolization if it is not identified and accounted for by using an alternatively sized device. Finally, the presence of excessive tissue from the Eustachian valve or the Chiari network in the RA may pose technical difficulty during the procedure in passage of the guidewire or interference with device positioning and deployment, resulting in malposition, residual leak, and/or embolization if not identified.

Atrial Septal Defect

In contrast to PFOs, ASDs are true deficiencies of tissue within the IAS. ASDs are present in 1 in 1500 live births[5] and are commonly diagnosed in adulthood when patients present with dyspnea, fatigue, atrial arrhythmias, and thromboembolic events. Although the small degree of shunting through a PFO is usually hemodynamically inconsequential (although right-to-left shunting may cause significant hypoxemia), the left-to-right shunt through an ASD can result in chronic right heart volume and pressure overload. Over time, RA and right ventricular (RV) dilatation and pulmonary hypertension may develop, although the latter to a milder degree than with higher pressure ventricular shunts. Symptoms often manifest as the LA and left ventricle become less compliant with age and, in turn, the degree of shunting increases. Eventually, the flow may become bidirectional as RA pressure rises over time, increasing the risk of paradoxic thromboembolic events.

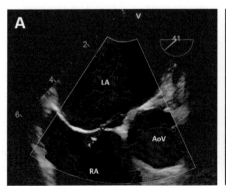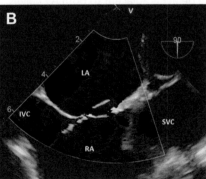

Fig. 2. PFO demonstrated by TEE in (A) basal short-axis and (B) bicaval views with color flow Doppler. AoV, aortic valve; SVC, superior vena cava.

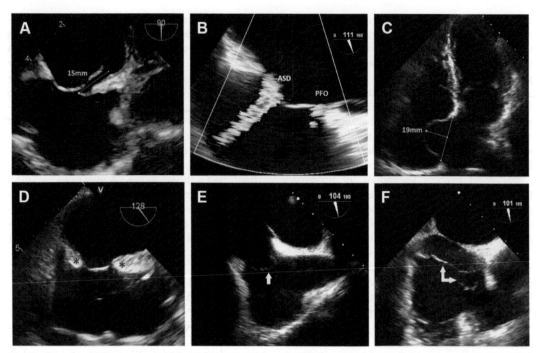

Fig. 3. Complex PFOs are those with (A) long tunnel lengths, (B) fenestrated or hybrid defects associated with ASDs, and those associated with (C) atrial septal aneurysms, (D) thickened septum secundum (asterisks), (E) prominent Eustachian valves (yellow arrow), or (F) extensive Chiari network (yellow arrows) that may pose technical challenges to percutaneous device closure.

ASDs are classified by the anatomic location and source of deficient atrial septal tissue (Fig. 4). An ostium secundum ASD is the most common form, about 75% of all ASDs,[5] and results from a defect of the septum primum. These defects are amenable to transcatheter closure if adequate rims are present. See later discussion of imaging characteristics of ostium secundum ASDs.

Ostium primum ASD is a defect in the inferior portion of the IAS resulting from abnormal fusion of the endocardial cushions and is, therefore, also called a partial or incomplete AV canal defect. The defect is adjacent to both AV valves, which are by definition abnormal in sharing a common AV annulus and valve plane. Percutaneous device closure is not possible because the septal defect is contiguous with the valve orifices and there is no AV rim.

Sinus venosus defects are located at the origin of the superior vena cava (SVC) or IVC, with absence of septal tissue between the vena cava and an adjacent pulmonary vein, resulting in a large left-to-right shunt. Concomitant partial anomalous pulmonary venous return (PAPVR) is frequently associated but is not necessary for the diagnosis. It is imperative to identify all pulmonary vein connections when the diagnosis of sinus venosus ASD is made. Sinus venosus ASDs should not be closed percutaneously because the lack of adequate rims predisposes to device embolization. In the setting of a sinus venosus ASD with PAPVR surgical baffles and reimplantation of the pulmonary veins are necessary.

The rarest form of ASD is the unroofed coronary sinus. This consists of a defect in the coronary sinus wall that drains from the coronary sinus os into the RA. This condition is commonly associated with a persistent left SVC. It is not amenable to transcatheter therapy.

DIAGNOSTIC IMAGING OF THE INTERATRIAL SEPTUM BY TRANSTHORACIC ECHOCARDIOGRAPHY

The initial imaging modality of choice for assessment of the IAS is TTE, a noninvasive, widely available technique without radiation exposure and with Doppler capabilities to assess the direction and degree of shunting. Beyond assessing the deficiency of the IAS itself, several other anatomic features should be evaluated in patients undergoing consideration for ASD closure. LA dimension and volume should be measured to stratify the risks of atrial arrhythmias and associated thromboembolism. Unexplained RA and RV

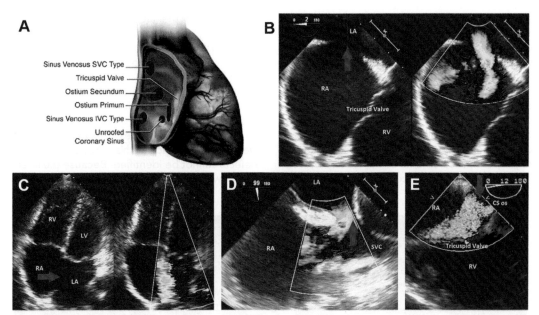

Fig. 4. Atrial septal defects are categorized by their location on the septum and the source of the deficient septal tissue. The defects are denoted by the red arrows. (*A*) Subtypes and locations of atrial septal defects as viewed from the RA. (*B*) Ostium secundum ASDs are the most common, approximately 75% of all ASDs, and are the most amenable to percutaneous device closure. (*C*) Ostium primum ASDs involve the AV valves and are, therefore, also called partial AV defects. (*D*) Superior or inferior sinus venosus ASDs are commonly associated with anomalous pulmonary vein returns. (*E*) The rarest of ASDs is unroofed coronary sinus that drains from the coronary sinus os into the RA. CS, coronary sinus; LV, left ventricle. (*From* Silvestry FE, Cohen MS, Armsby LB, et al. Guidelines for the echocardiographic assessment of atrial septal defect and patent foramen ovale: from the American Society of Echocardiography and Society for Cardiac Angiography and Interventions. J Am Soc Echocardiogr 2015;28(8):912; with permission from Elsevier.)

dilatation warrants a close evaluation for septal defects. The American College of Cardiology (ACC)/American Heart Association (AHA) guidelines provide a class I recommendation for ASD closure if RA and RV dilatation is identified with or without concomitant symptoms (level of evidence B).[6] RV remodeling does not typically occur due to shunting from a PFO alone. Pulmonary artery systolic pressure (PASP) should be measured to assess for the presence of pulmonary hypertension. Pulmonary artery dilatation, RV hypertrophy, leftward septal shift, and bidirectional or right-to-left shunt are suggestive of significant pulmonary hypertension, which, if severe and irreversible, is a contraindication to closure. In regard to the permissible degree of pulmonary hypertension, the ACC/AHA guidelines state that closure of an ASD, either percutaneously or surgically, may be considered in the presence of net left-to-right shunting, pulmonary artery pressure less than two-thirds systemic levels, pulmonary vascular resistance less than two-thirds systemic vascular resistance, or when responsive to either pulmonary vasodilator therapy or test occlusion of the defect (class IIb, level of evidence C).[6]

The presence of significant left ventricular dysfunction or echocardiographic evidence of elevated left ventricular end diastolic pressure (LVEDP) must be considered before device closure because sudden occlusion of the shunt without appropriate diuresis may increase left-sided pressures and precipitate heart failure. Test-occlusion during the procedure with measurement of LVEDP may be helpful in these cases.

TTE is rarely able to visualize the anatomic detail of a PFO; rather, the presence of a PFO is suggested by color flow Doppler and agitated saline study. By contrast, an ASD shunt can usually be seen by both 2D imaging and color flow Doppler. Multiple views by TTE are necessary to characterize the size, shape, and location of the defect with specific attention to the neighboring structures and tissue rims. The length of available rims between the defect to the vena cava, pulmonary veins, coronary sinus, aorta, and the mitral and tricuspid valves is critical to determining whether the anatomy is suitable for percutaneous closure. In children, TTE is often adequate for full ASD assessment. However, in adults, the IAS is a relatively posterior structure that is more distant from the transthoracic probe, and TEE should be performed to provide a complete evaluation. If a TEE is not possible (eg, patient comorbidities, swallowing difficulties, esophageal disease), the PFO or ASD can be interrogated with ICE before defect closure (see later discussion). The lower rim adjacent to the IVC may be particularly challenging to image, especially after device placement due to shadowing. In general, one should avoid relying on measurements of defect size by TTE. Artifactual dropout is common with the thin septum when the ultrasound beam is parallel to the IAS, as is the case in apical 4-chamber and parasternal short-axis (SAX) windows.

The subcostal view provides the optimal imaging window because the ultrasound beam is orthogonal to the plane of the IAS (Fig. 5). The subcostal 4-chamber view demonstrates the anterior-posterior axis of IAS, from the posterior atrial roof to the AV valves. The vena cava is not well visualized, and, in this view, sinus venosus defects cannot be identified. Because the interatrial flow through the ASD is now parallel to the

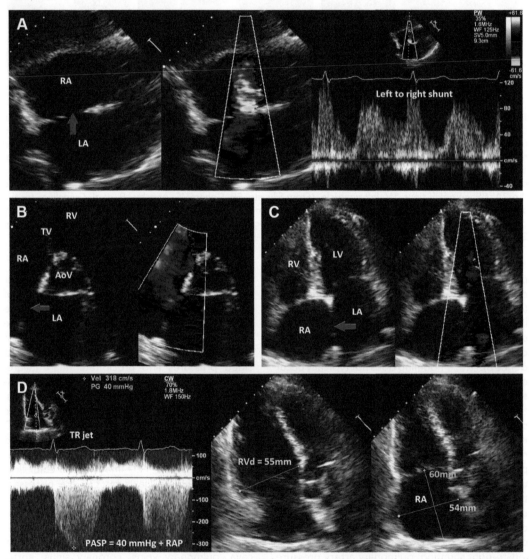

Fig. 5. Common TTE windows used to evaluate the IAS for ASD and PFO. The defects are denoted by the red arrows. (A) Subcostal frontal view with ultrasound beam orthogonal to the IAS plane. Shunt flow direction is parallel to the beam and is interrogated with color flow and pulsed wave Doppler. (B) Parasternal basal short axis visualizes the anterior-posterior axis of the septum. (C) The apical 4-chamber view provides (D) hemodynamic assessment with measurements of the RA and RV dimensions and PASP by the tricuspid regurgitation jet. RAP, RA pressure; RVd, RV dimension; TR, tricuspid regurgitation; TV, tricuspid valve.

ultrasound beam, color flow, pulsed wave (PW), and continuous wave (CW) Doppler can be used to determine shunt direction and pressure gradient. Tilting the probe rightward toward the liver can bring the IVC and any inferior sinus venosus defect into view. Turning the transducer 90° counterclockwise for the subcostal sagittal view visualizes the superior-inferior axis of the IAS with the SVC and IVC coming into view with a slight rightward tilt of the probe. In this bicaval view, superior sinus venosus defects can be identified. Alternatively, the right parasternal window also offers a bicaval view with the SVC in the near field adjacent to the right upper pulmonary vein (RUPV) with the right pulmonary artery visible in cross-section. The parasternal SAX window at the base of the heart provides the anterior-posterior view, identifying the aortic and posterior rims to the defect. The apical 4-chamber view visualizes the length of the IAS to the AV valves and can be used to diagnose primum ASDs. This is also the view from which RA and RV chamber sizes are measured and PASP is estimated from the tricuspid regurgitation jet to provide an assessment of the hemodynamic impact of the ASD. This window is also frequently used for agitated saline contrast study for the identification of a PFO.

Agitated Saline Contrast Study

Color Doppler flow on TTE is insensitive (28%) but highly specific (100%) for the detection of a PFO.[7] Agitated saline contrast study improves the sensitivity of PFO detection by TTE. The sensitivity is improved only modestly by agitated saline injection alone (sensitivity 58%, specificity 98%).[7] Provocative maneuvers, such as the Valsalva maneuver, sniff, or cough, transiently increase venous return and RA pressure to enhance right-to-left shunting. Adequate provocation is manifest by leftward bowing of the IAS to indicate elevated RA pressure. Notably, it is during the release of the Valsalva maneuver that the venous return and RA pressure increase.[8] The use of saline contrast with provocative maneuvers improves the sensitivity of PFO detection substantially to 99% with 5 attempts (95% with 1 attempt) but with a concomitant decrease in specificity (85%). False-negative tests can occur with elevated LA pressures and inadequate provocative maneuvers.

An effective agitated saline injection fully opacifies the RA wall adjacent to the IAS, with a long loop of at least 10 seconds recorded to visualize the crossing of bubbles. Any window in which the anterior-superior aspect of the IAS and the RA-LA junction can be well visualized

can be used. The apical 4-chamber (Fig. 6), basal parasternal SAX, and subcostal 4-chamber views are most commonly used. Biplane can be used to increase detection sensitivity for small shunts. Early microbubbles seen within 3 to 6 cardiac cycles suggest intracardiac shunt and constitute a positive study. Late microbubbles are consistent with intrapulmonary or extracardiac shunts such as arterial-venous malformations.

PREPROCEDURAL IMAGING OF ATRIAL SEPTAL DEFECTS AND PATENT FORAMEN OVALE WITH TRANSESOPHAGEAL ECHOCARDIOGRAPHY

If an ASD or PFO is identified on TTE, or if the agitated saline study is positive, a TEE should be performed to better visualize the anatomy of the defect and determine suitability for percutaneous device closure. TEE is also indicated if the clinical suspicion for interatrial shunt or cardioembolic source remains high despite a negative TTE (eg, increased right-sided volumes). Before any percutaneous intervention, defining the dimensions and features of the defect and its surrounding structures is essential to determining anatomic suitability and device selection.

Patent Foramen Ovale Assessment by Transesophageal Echocardiography

The septum primum flap can be visualized in the superior-inferior axis using the bicaval view

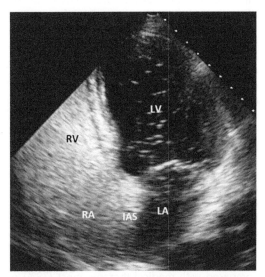

Fig. 6. Agitated saline contrast study for PFO detection. Effective saline injection fully opacifies the RA wall adjacent to the IAS. Early microbubbles within 3 to 6 cardiac cycles constitute a positive study for intracardiac shunt.

(midesophageal [ME] window at approximately 90°–120°) and the anterior-posterior axis in the basal SAX view (ME window at approximately 30°–75°) (see Fig. 2). The presence of an ASA or a thickened septum secundum should be noted because this may affect the stability and position of the occluder device and influence device size selection. Hybrid defects with an associated ASD that may be distant from the PFO should also be identified because these will generally need to be closed if the indication for PFO closure is stroke or hypoxemia. The ACC/AHA guidelines state that closure of an ASD is reasonable in the presence of paradoxic embolism or documented orthodeoxia-platypnea (class IIa, level of evidence C and B, respectively).[6] The tunnel length, as determined by the orifice size to both the RA and LA, and associated defects or fenestrations should be identified and measured (see Fig. 3).

Given the location of the PFO at the anterior-superior edge of the fossa ovalis, the historical approach to sizing Amplatzer-type devices used the minimal distance from the PFO to aorta anteriorly and from the PFO to SVC superiorly to determine device eligibility and selection. However, a study from the Mayo Clinic reported that 66% of autopsied normal hearts would have been ineligible for the smallest devices based on minimal distance requirements.[9] The sizes of occluder devices used for PFO closure are defined by the diameter of the RA disc (Amplatzer PFO Occluder, St. Jude Medical, Minneapolis, MN, USA) or the diameter of the 2 equal-sized discs (Amplatzer Multifenestrated Occluder, St. Jude Medical, Minneapolis, MN, USA; and Cardioform Septal Occluder, WL Gore, Flagstaff, AZ, USA). Most operators select the appropriate device size by doubling the distance of either the stretched balloon diameter (on fluoroscopy, TEE, or ICE) or the distance between the inferior edge of the PFO to the septum secundum superiorly when the PFO is propped open by a stiff exchange wire. In the absence of complex anatomy (ie, an ASA or thick septum secundum), some operators simply choose a default size (ie, 25 mm). In the Recurrent Stroke Comparing PFO Closure to Established Current Standard of Care Treatment (RESPECT) randomized clinical trial, which demonstrated the safety and efficacy of PFO closure with the Amplatzer PFO Occluder compared with medical therapy, most (79%) of the subjects received a 25 mm device[10,11] although the historical sizing method was recommended (but not required) by the study protocol. The occurrence of cardiac erosion is

exceedingly rare after PFO closure, irrespective of small rims. In the RESPECT trial, there were no cases of device erosion, even at an average of 6-year follow-up. Erosions have not been reported to date with the Cardioform Septal Occluder.

Atrial Septal Defect Assessment by Transesophageal Echocardiography

The shape and size of the defect, the presence and lengths of tissue rims, and the presence of multiple defects or fenestrations must be carefully assessed to determine device eligibility, as well as sizing (Box 1). Color flow, PW, and CW Doppler can be used when the septum is orthogonal to the ultrasound beam, such as in the bicaval or basal SAX views. The presence of fenestrations or multiple defects may require larger

---

Box 1
Characteristics of atrial septal defect to be measured and reported by transthoracic echocardiography and transesophageal echocardiography

ASD type: PFO, primum ASD, secundum ASD, or other atrial communication (sinus venosus defect, unroofed coronary sinus, anomalous pulmonary vein drainage)

Doppler flow: presence of left to right, right to left or bidirectional flow

Presence or absence of ASA

Associated findings: eustachian valve or Chiari network

ASD size: maximal and minimal diameters (optimally measured from 3D volume data sets), ASD area

ASD location in septum (high secundum ASD, sinus venosus defect SVC, or IVC type)

Measurement of all rims: aortic, RUPV, superior, posterior, inferior, AV septal

Shape of ASD: round, oval, irregular

Presence of multiple fenestrations

Dynamic nature of ASD: measurement of area and maximum-minimal diameters in end-systole and end-diastole

Stop-flow diameter of ASD (when balloon sizing is used for percutaneous transcatheter closure)

From Silvestry FE, Cohen MS, Armsby LB, et al. Guidelines for the echocardiographic assessment of atrial septal defect and patent foramen ovale: from the American Society of Echocardiography and Society for Cardiac Angiography and Interventions. J Am Soc Echocardiogr 2015;28(8):944; with permission from Elsevier.

or multiple devices, or a dedicated device for multifenestrated defects for effective closure. ASDs can be round, elliptical, or slit-like. The maximal ASD diameter is first measured in standard 2D TEE planes. Measurements should be obtained in both systole and diastole, with dynamic ASD being defined by at least a 50% change in dimension over a cardiac cycle. In general, the device size is dictated by its maximal linear dimension in diastole (although some operators have proposed using a mean diameter for Amplatzer-type devices). Many operators decide on a final device size by slowly inflating a sizing balloon during the procedure while interrogating the defect with simultaneous color Doppler; the diameter of the defect is then defined as the diameter of the balloon when color flow ceases completely (the stop-flow diameter).

The tissue rims around the ASD should be identified and measured. Moving clockwise from the superior aspect, the 5 standard rims as seen from the RA are: superior, anterior-superior, anterior-inferior, posterior-inferior,

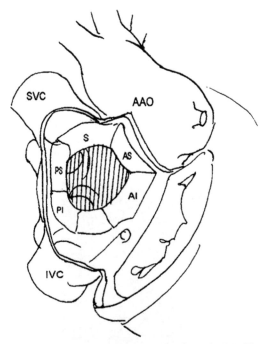

Fig. 7. Interatrial septal rims as seen from the RA. The 5 standard rims are the SVC superiorly (S), anterior-superior (AS) aortic root and ascending aorta (AAO), anterior-inferior (AI) tricuspid valve, the posterior-inferior (PI) IVC, and the posterior-superior (PS) free wall. (*From* Mathewson JW, Bichell D, Rothman A, et al. Absent posteroinferior and anterosuperior atrial septal defect rims: Factors affecting nonsurgical closure of large secundum defects using the Amplatzer occluder. J Am Soc Echocardiogr 2004;17(1):63; with permission from Elsevier.)

and posterior (Fig. 7). These rims can also be described using a simplified nomenclature: the SVC rim, the aortic (or retroaortic) rim, the AV rim, the IVC rim, and the posterior rim. Deficient rims are defined as less than 5 mm.

Most views of the IAS are obtained at the ME level.[2,12] The anterior-posterior dimension of the defect, as well as the anterior-superior aortic rim and posterior rim, can be measured from the basal SAX at the level of the aortic valve (ME 30°–75°). The superior-inferior dimension and the SVC and IVC rims can be seen in the bicaval view (ME 90°–120°) (Fig. 8). A superior sinus venosus ASD can be identified in this view. If the IVC rim is not adequately visualized in the bicaval view, retroflexion and/or slowly decreasing the omniplane probe angle to 60° can bring the IVC into view. An inferior sinus venosus ASD can be visualized in this window. Increasing the probe omniplane angle by 10° to 20° brings the coronary sinus into view immediately adjacent to the IVC, separated by the Eustachian valve. Slight clockwise rotation of the probe brings the RUPV into view in front of the SVC (Fig. 9). The deep transgastric window can also provide a sagittal bicaval view by first identifying the RV inflow view at 90° and increasing the omniplane angle to approximately 100° to 120° with slight clockwise rotation of the probe (see Fig. 8).

All 4 pulmonary veins should be identified, especially if sinus venosus ASD is diagnosed and associated PAPVR is suspected. PAPVR can also occur with ostium secundum ASDs, although this is less common. The left upper pulmonary vein (LUPV) is immediately lateral to the left atrial appendage (LAA), separated by the limbus or Coumadin ridge. The LUPV can be identified by withdrawing the probe slightly and rotating counterclockwise from ME 40° to 60° adjacent to the LAA. The left lower pulmonary vein (LLPV) can be found adjacent to the LUPV by advancing the probe slightly and rotating further counterclockwise. Alternatively, the bifurcation of LUPV and LLPV can be located by withdrawing the probe to the upper esophagus, centering the image on LUPV, and increasing the omniplane angle to 90° to 100°. Clockwise rotation toward the patient's right brings the bifurcation of the right pulmonary veins and cross-section of the right pulmonary artery into view (see Fig. 9). If all 4 pulmonary veins cannot be identified, computed tomography scanning with contrast should be performed to exclude PAPVR before device closure.

Finally, the 4-chamber (ME 0°–30°) view defines the defect's relationship to the AV valves with the anterior-inferior rim to the tricuspid

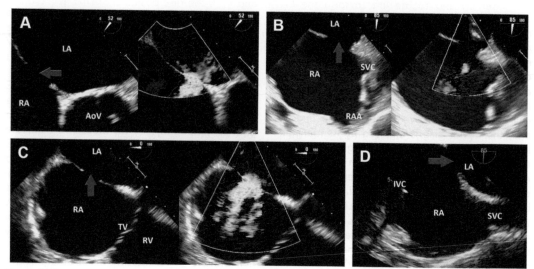

Fig. 8. TEE assessment of the IAS. Basic 2D views of the IAS are obtained from ME windows with (A) the basal SAX (ME 30°–75°) visualizing the anterior-posterior axis, (B) the bicaval view (ME 90°–120°) visualizing the superior-inferior axis, and (C) the 4-chamber view (ME 0°–30°) defining the anterior-inferior AV rim. (D) Alternative sagittal bicaval view can be obtained from the deep transgastric window by increasing the omniplane angle from the RV inflow view at 90° to approximately 100° to 110°. The defects are denoted by the red arrows. RAA, RA appendage.

and mitral valves (see Fig. 8). Primum ASDs can be identified in this view. However, because the ultrasound beam is parallel to the IAS in the 4-chamber view and artifactual drop-out can occur, clockwise rotation toward the RA can place the beam orthogonal to the plane of the IAS and allow a more reliable measurement. Finally, withdrawing the probe to the upper esophagus at 0° to 30° provides the basal transverse view that depicts the relationship of the ASD to the SVC, RUPV, and ascending aorta.

Three-Dimensional Transesophageal Echocardiography Assessment of the Interatrial Septum

Advances in ultrasound and computing technology have moved beyond multiplane 2D imaging to high-resolution 3D real-time imaging. Comprehensive 3D TEE produces more complete depictions of the defect and its relationship to surrounding structures. The 3D image can be acquired in narrow-sector real-time, wide-sector zoomed, or full-volume gated

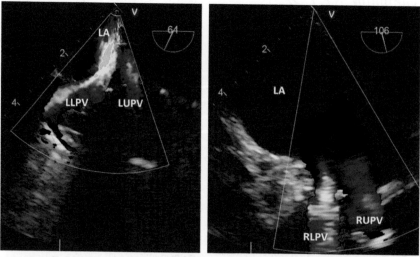

Fig. 9. TEE identification of the pulmonary veins. All 4 pulmonary veins should be identified when an ASD is diagnosed because anomalous pulmonary vein returns are frequently associated with sinus venosus ASDs. LLPV, left lower pulmonary vein; LUPV, left upper pulmonary vein; RLPV, right lower pulmonary vein; RUPV, right upper pulmonary vein.

acquisition over multiple cardiac cycles.[13] Each mode has benefits and drawbacks in balancing temporal and spatial resolution while optimizing the conditions to avoid imaging artifacts. Stitching artifact from gated acquisition is common with irregular rhythms or from respiratory motion. The 3D acquisition is obtained from standard 2D views, such as the basal aortic SAX or bicaval view of the IAS. The 2D image should be optimized before 3D acquisition. Gain settings should be optimized at the time of acquisition to avoid artifactual drop-out that may falsely appear to be multiple defects, which cannot be recovered in postprocessing.

These stored 3D datasets can be manipulated in real-time or off-line for orientation and measurements. The 3D image can be cropped, oriented, and reconstructed before measurements are obtained. Cropping at the time of acquisition reduces the sector of interest to improve spatial and temporal resolution but cannot be uncropped after acquisition. Importantly, in contrast to cross-sectional viewing of most radiographic modalities, 3D echocardiography requires cropping of the overlying structures to reveal the structure of interest *en face*.

The IAS and defect are then rotated to orient to the standard anatomic convention of viewing the septum from the RA and aligning the SVC-IVC along the vertical axis and aorta anteriorly toward the upper right of the image (Fig. 10).[2,14] To view from the LA side, the 3D image is flipped along its superior-inferior axis like opening a book. From the LA perspective, the RUPV is adjacent to the SVC in the superior position, the aortic root is anterior-superior toward the upper left of the image, and the mitral valve is anterior-inferior. The final step is to perform multiplanar reconstruction (MPR). Two axes are placed along the major and minor axes of the defect along the IAS, and the third axis is orthogonal to the plane of the septum (Fig. 11). The planes are moved and tilted to align the defect and rims in each MPR viewing panel. The maximal size of the ASD and the surrounding rims can then be measured on a true cross-sectional 2D plane at end-diastole. After device deployment, the same views and MPR can be used to determine whether the device fully covers the defect, is stably seated on the septum, and is not interacting in a harmful way with any of its surrounding structures.

INTRAPROCEDURAL ECHOCARDIOGRAPHIC GUIDANCE FOR TRANSCATHETER DEVICE CLOSURE OF ATRIAL SEPTAL DEFECT AND PATENT FORAMEN OVALE

Real-time echocardiography is used in conjunction with fluoroscopy to provide procedural guidance during percutaneous device closure and monitor for complications during and after the procedure. TTE is the least invasive and may provide adequate visualization in pediatric patients but adults usually require TEE or ICE for intraprocedural imaging. TEE provides excellent imaging quality with the advantage of real-time 3D imaging to comprehensively assess the defect and its surrounding structures from various perspectives before and after device placement. The primary disadvantages of intraprocedural TEE are the need for anesthesia support and a dedicated echocardiographer.

For these reasons, ICE has become an attractive alternative for intraprocedural imaging. Conscious sedation is adequate for ICE, reducing the risk and duration of the procedure. The

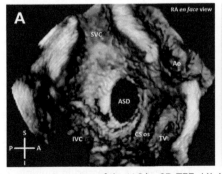
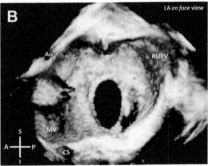

Fig. 10. Anatomic orientation of the IAS by 3D TEE. (A) Anatomic orientation of the IAS follows the convention of viewing the septum *en face* from the RA and aligning the SVC and IVC along the superior-inferior axis and the aorta anterior-superiorly toward the upper right. (B) The left atrial *en face* perspective of the septum can be obtained by turning the 3D image along its superior-inferior axis like opening a book. The RUPV is visible adjacent to the SVC. MV, mitral valve.

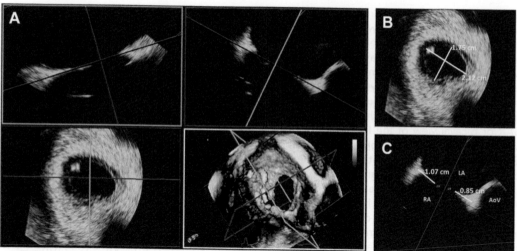

Fig. 11. Multiplanar reconstruction of ASD from 3D TEE. (A) Three mutually orthogonal axes are oriented to the septal defect to create the plane of the IAS (lower left panel with the blue border) and 2 intersecting perpendicular planes. Note that the planes on the 3D representation may not visually align as they appear on the 2D images due to the parallax effect. (B) The major and minor axes of the septal defect and (C) the rims (the posterior and aortic rims) are measured.

imaging quality is excellent and comparable to TEE. The interventionalist manipulates the ICE catheter and obviates the need for a dedicated imager. However, ICE is invasive, requiring an 8 to 11F venous catheter for the single-use ultrasound. The far field views are relatively limited when imaging from the RA, and wide-angle 3D ICE imaging is not yet routinely available, although they are in development.[2,15,16]

Transesophageal Echocardiographic Guidance of Device Closure

As previously described for preprocedural TEE assessment of the IAS, the defect and its surrounding rims are measured for device selection and sizing. Real-time 3D imaging can be used to complement 2D views throughout the procedure to verify the position, orientation, and stability of the device and its relationship to neighboring structures. In addition, 2D biplane imaging can provide simultaneous visualization of 2 orthogonal planes, such as the basal SAX and the bicaval views, at a higher temporal resolution (frame rate) than 3D allows and can be particularly useful for real-time procedural guidance.

Venous access is typically obtained via the IVC and can be visualized in the bicaval view as the guide wire is directed superiorly and toward the IAS to enter the LA via the defect. The wire should be visualized in the RA to avoid entry into the RA appendage adjacent to the SVC, a potential site for atrial perforation. It is also important to note the presence of a Chiari network because there is a risk for wire entanglement and complex maneuvers in the RA should be avoided. Occasionally, the operator might find crossing the PFO with the wire challenging due to the orientation of the IAS relative to the IVC. In these cases, the echocardiographer can help direct the wire and catheter into the fossa ovalis.

After passage into the LA, the wire and the delivery sheath are advanced posteriorly into the LUPV, a safe structure in which to park the delivery apparatus. Echocardiographic imaging can guide and confirm the passage of the wire in the LUPV and away from the LAA, a thin-walled trabeculated structure at risk for perforation (Fig. 12). Next, the delivery sheath is repositioned into the LA body and the LA disc is deployed under echocardiographic visualization to ensure that the device is away from the LAA, the mitral valve, and the atrial free wall. The LA disc is pulled into position adjacent to the IAS at the defect while the connecting waist is deployed with continuing traction toward the RA. Finally, the RA disc is deployed on the RA aspect of the IAS and cinches closed the defect. With Amplatzer-type devices, a tug test can be performed and should be monitored by echocardiography and fluoroscopy to ensure stability.

The device is assessed in multiple 2D and 3D views to verify that the RA and LA discs are in their respective chambers. The position of the device and the presence of tissue between the discs, indicated by slight separation of the discs

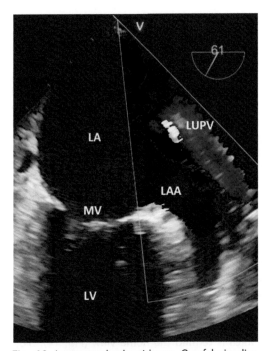

Fig. 12. Intraprocedural guidance. Careful visualization of the wire and delivery sheath toward the LUPV while avoiding the adjacent LAA, a thin-walled structure at risk of perforation.

in profile, should be confirmed in both 2D and 3D (Fig. 13). The device and surrounding rims should be interrogated by color flow Doppler to assess for any residual shunts. If uncertainty remains about whether a full seal was achieved, agitated saline contrast study can be performed as previously described. Small shunts will often decrease or resolve as the device endothelializes over a few months, but residual shunts persist in 3% at 1 year postimplantation.[17]

In many cases, shunting will be identified along the retroaortic rim after device deployment but before device release. This is due to tension from the delivery cable tugging the RA disc inferiorly away from the septum. This tension and flow will resolve after device release from the delivery cable, but the operator should make sure that the residual leak is not from an undersized device or from the device slipping from the LA into the RA at the site of a deficient retroaortic rim. For residual shunting during follow-up or if new symptoms develop, the device should be interrogated by TEE to assess for new or worsening shunt and to determine whether a repeat procedure to seal the leak is warranted.

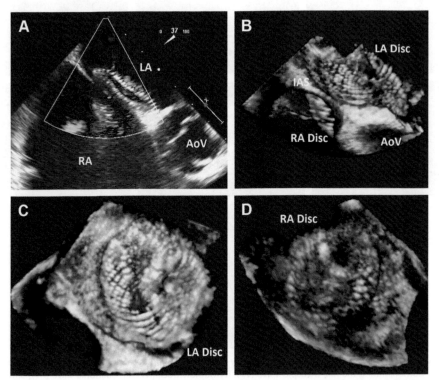

Fig. 13. Intraprocedural guidance of ASD closure device deployment. The delivery sheath is placed in the body of the LA; and the LA disc, the waist, and the RA disc are sequentially deployed under echocardiographic and fluoroscopic visualization. Full assessment of the device and the surrounding tissue is performed in (A) 2D and (B) 3D to visualize the (C) LA and (D) RA discs of the closure device.

Neighboring structures, including the aortic root, the mitral and tricuspid valves, the coronary sinus, the pulmonary veins, the SVC, and the IVC, should be assessed to ensure that there is no impingement or deformation before the release of the device. The mitral and tricuspid valves should be interrogated with color flow and CW Doppler to assess for valvular regurgitation and stenosis. It is important to reiterate that the closure device is under tension from the delivery system until released, and the final conformation of the device and septum may change slightly when fully released. Nevertheless, echocardiographic assessment must be performed before release to permit opportunity for recapture and repositioning.

Intracardiac Echocardiography

ICE plays an important role in procedural guidance of PFO and ASD closure, and has several advantages compared with TEE. Intraprocedural ICE obviates general anesthesia and a dedicated echocardiographer. In doing so, ICE improves patient comfort, allows for rapid postprocedure recovery, improves catheterization laboratory efficiency and turn-over times, and reduces resource utilization. ICE imaging also allows for same-day discharge after closure in appropriate patients.[18] ICE can identify all the rims required for transcatheter ASD closure, is highly sensitive in detecting a interatrial shunt by agitated saline study, and can provide excellent imaging of the inferior septum (the IVC rim), which can be challenging to assess by TEE.[19] A prospective, 1000 subject, 2-center study demonstrated that ICE-guided PFO closure was safe and associated with high rates of procedural success.[20]

Technical approach to intracardiac imaging for patent foramen ovale or atrial septal defect closure

The ICE catheter is advanced through the femoral vein into the low RA. The catheter should be rotated clockwise until the tricuspid valve, RV, and RV outflow tract are visualized, which is termed the home view (Fig. 14). Slow

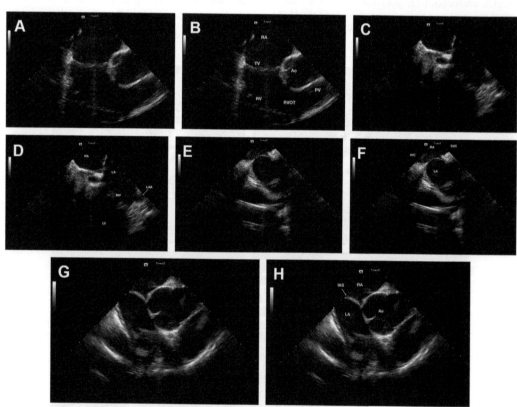

Fig. 14. Fundamentals of intracardiac echocardiography (ICE) imaging of the IAS for PFO and ASD closure. (*A, B*) The home view, demonstrating the RA, tricuspid valve (TV), RV outflow track (RVOT), pulmonic valve (PV), and aorta (Ao). (*C, D*) Clockwise rotation of the ICE catheter brings into view the left-sided cardiac structures: the LA, MV, LAA, and LV. (*E, F*) Further clockwise rotation of the catheter until the IAS is visualized, followed by posterior flexion of the catheter tip, demonstrates the long-axis of the IAS and fossa ovalis. (*G, H*) The catheter is clocked further (while maintaining posterior flexion) to reveal the SAX view, identified by the 3 leaflets of the aortic valve (IAS, interatrial septum; Ao, aorta).

clockwise rotation of the catheter will then bring the mitral valve into view. The operator should continue to rotate the catheter clockwise until the mitral valve disappears from view and the IAS appears at the top of the image. At this point, the operator should advance the catheter slightly and flex the catheter-tip posteriorly using the appropriate actuator knob. This will reveal the IAS in its long axis. Occasionally, slight flexing of the tip in the left direction will provide a more complete view of this structure. The catheter should be advanced (toward the SVC) to image the superior aspect of the septum and withdrawn (toward the IVC) to assess the inferior septum. Often, the long-axis view of the IAS is optimal for an agitated saline injection to confirm the presence of a PFO. From the long-axis view, the SAX of the IAS can be obtained by either rotating the entire catheter further clockwise or by flexing the catheter tip aggressively to the left until the 3 leaflets of the aortic valve or the aortic root are visualized. The SAX view is usually the optimal one to guide implantation of the occluder device in the setting of an ASD with deficient retroaortic rim. Fluoroscopy can assist in positioning the ICE catheter if acquiring the correct image is difficult (Fig. 15).

Key intracardiac echocardiography assessments after device implantation
After device deployment, ICE should be used to confirm that the device is in an adequate and stable position. First, each disc of the device should be in its appropriate chamber, without prolapse of both discs of the device into the RA or LA. This can be accomplished with the long-axis

view (superior and inferior rims) and the short-axis view (retroaortic and posterior rims). If there is any question about whether the septal tissue has been sandwiched between the left and right discs, this can be clarified by tugging on the delivery cable while visualizing the septum on ICE and confirming that the septum is between the discs. Advancing and withdrawing the ICE catheter will allow the operator to interrogate the superior and inferior aspects of the device, respectively. The area around the device should be interrogated with color flow Doppler to identify any residual leak that might require device recapture and repositioning, upsizing, or the implantation of a second device.

In the case of PFO closure, the operator should confirm that the RA disc splays over the septum secundum and does not fall within the PFO tunnel (Fig. 16). If that is indeed the case, either the RA disc should be recaptured and redeployed with greater tension on the LA disc against the septum, or the device should be removed and a larger size selected. Finally, after device release, an agitated saline study can be performed to confirm that the right-to-left shunt through the PFO has been abrogated, although it is not uncommon for a small residual leak to be present acutely that will close over weeks to months after the device endothelializes.[21]

ASSESSING FOR COMPLICATIONS OF ATRIAL SEPTAL DEFECT AND PATENT FORAMEN OVALE CLOSURE

A key role for echocardiographic guidance is to monitor real-time for procedural complications.

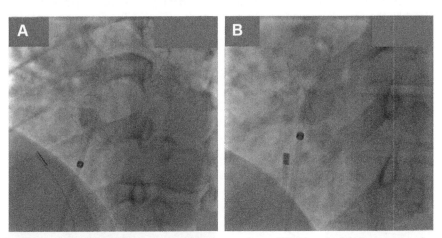

Fig. 15. Fluoroscopy of key ICE catheter positions for transcatheter PFO closure. (*A*) The imaging element of the ICE catheter is directed up and to the right of the screen in the anterior-posterior projection when imaging the long-axis of the IAS. This position is obtained by advancing the ICE catheter from the right femoral vein into the low-to-mid RA, rotating clockwise, and flexing the catheter tip posteriorly. (*B*) The ICE catheter has been rotated clockwise approximately 60° to 90° from its position in panel A to image the basal short axis of the IAS.

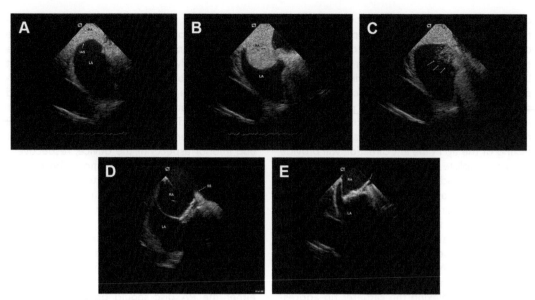

Fig. 16. ICE-guided transcatheter PFO closure in a cryptogenic stroke patient. (A) Agitated saline injection fills the RA in a cryptogenic stroke patient with obstructive sleep apnea undergoing ICE-guided transcatheter PFO closure. (B) Profound excursion of the IAS toward the LA occurs during respiration. (C) After this excursion, bubbles are seen transiting from the RA to LA through the PFO (arrows). (D) A Helex Septal Occluder 25 mm device (W.L. Gore, Flagstaff, AZ, USA) was deployed. ICE imaging demonstrates that during snoring the superior portion of the RA disc falls off the septum secundum (arrow). (E) The device is recaptured, and a 30 mm device was deployed successfully. ICE imaging demonstrates that the RA disc is splayed over the septum secundum (arrow). SS, septum secundum.

The immediate risk of any intracardiac procedure is cardiac trauma and perforation resulting in pericardial effusion and tamponade. At the start of the procedure, it is critical to obtain baseline imaging of the pericardial contour and the presence of any pericardial effusion, even if trivial, as a comparison point for any intraprocedural changes. The atria and the atrial appendages are thinwalled structures that are prone to perforation.[17,22] Notably, the septum secundum rim of the IAS is an infolding of atrial tissue and is, therefore, contiguous with the outside of the heart. Perforation or erosion through the septum secundum via the posterior free wall may result in pericardial effusion and tamponade. Similarly, the aortic root is immediately adjacent to the anterior aspect between the 2 atria with pericardial tissue reflected on it, creating the transverse sinus, another high-risk area for perforation and tamponade (Fig. 17). Frequent imaging of the

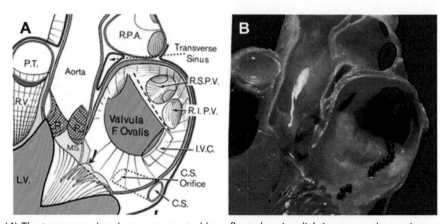

Fig. 17. (A) The transverse sinus is a space created by reflected pericardial tissue over the aortic root anteriorly between the 2 atria. (B) It is a high-risk area for device erosion and cardiac perforation. (From Amin Z. Echocardiographic predictors of cardiac erosion after Amplatzer septal occluder placement. Catheter Cardiovasc Interv 2014;83(1):87; with permission from Wiley.)

pericardium after each major maneuver of the delivery sheath, after device deployment, and with any unexpected hemodynamic perturbation is imperative for rapid identification and immediate response to a traumatic pericardial effusion. A TTE within 24 hours postprocedure is recommended both to confirm device placement and to reassess the pericardial space for effusion. The presence of a pericardial effusion after Amplatzer Septal Occluder implantation has been associated with the presence of device erosion.

The development of thrombus on the delivery apparatus or the closure device should also be monitored. Thrombus within the LA or LAA is a contraindication to proceeding and should be ruled out before the start of the procedure. Device thrombus rarely occurs over follow-up. In a series of 1000 subjects who received a range of occluder devices for ASD and PFO closure and underwent surveillance TEE at 4 weeks and 6 months postprocedure, device thrombus was identified in approximately 2% of cases.[23] Device thrombus was most frequent with occluders no longer in clinical use, and it was quite uncommon with Amplatzer devices (0%) and the Helex device (0.8%). Reported risk factors for thrombus formation after device closure include the presence of atrial fibrillation, persistent ASA, and noncompliance with antiplatelet agents before the device is fully endothelialized. Most occur within the first month after device implantation and are identified by TEE rather than TTE. Most occurrences resolve with anticoagulation.[17,23] Many operators do not reverse heparin anticoagulation with protamine postprocedure to avoid any diathesis toward device thrombus formation.

Device embolization is a rare but serious occurrence (0.1%–0.4%) that can occur immediately after release or weeks to months later and requires percutaneous or surgical retrieval.[2,24] Embolization typically results from undersized device, deficient or floppy rims not taken into account with device sizing, or malpositioning. Visualization of any movement or prolapse of the device during the tug test can alert the interventionalist to device instability and provide opportunity to reposition or replace with a larger device before device release.

Echocardiographic Predictors of Device Erosion

Device erosion is a rare but potentially catastrophic complication (0.1%–0.3%) that came to attention through safety reporting after the initial pivotal studies of ASD closure with Amplatzer devices.[2,25–28] Almost all occurred within 3 months

of implantation, with a significant number within the first week. However, rare occurrences up to 3 years after device implantation have been reported. Most required surgical repair and device removal. The isolated mortality rate of 0.05% with transcatheter closure, even accounting for erosion, remains well below the estimated surgical mortality of 0.13% based on Society of Thoracic Surgeons score.[27] Device erosions are exceedingly rare after PFO closure, occurring in 0.02% of 11,000 patients in the manufacturer AGA registry,[22] and occurring in none of the patients enrolled in the RESPECT clinical trial.[10] Erosions have not been reported to date with the Helex or Cardioform devices, although strut fractures have been identified during follow-up with the former.

Several studies reviewed the cases of erosion and identified echocardiographic features that were more common among those who later had device erosions, although the absolute risk remains low even with the presence of these features (**Box 2**).[17,25,26,29] In an early study, 90% of defects with erosion had deficient retroaortic (anterior-superior) rim and/or a high ASD with deficient superior rim with erosion involving the aortic root or atrial roof.[26] Interestingly, absent

---

Box 2
Echocardiographic features associated with device erosion

Deficient aortic rim in multiple views, absent aortic rim at 0° (bald aorta)

Deficient superior rim in multiple views

Superior location of secundum ASD

Oversized ASD device (device diameter >1.5 times static stop-flow diameter)

Dynamic ASD (50% change in size of ASD)

Use of 26-mm ASO device

Malaligned defect

Tenting of atrial septal free wall after placement of device (into transverse sinus)

Wedging of device disc between posterior wall and aorta

Pericardial effusion present after device placement

From Silvestry FE, Cohen MS, Armsby LB, et al. Guidelines for the echocardiographic assessment of atrial septal defect and patent foramen ovale: from the American Society of Echocardiography and Society for Cardiac Angiography and Interventions. J Am Soc Echocardiogr 2015;28(8):947; with permission from Elsevier.

retroaortic rim is common and has been reported in almost half of ASDs, yet erosions are quite rare.[30] Further analysis of the erosion cases found that the retroaortic rim was deficient in more than 1 TEE SAX view (eg, 20°, 30°, 40°), indicating that the rim was deficient for a substantial circumference of the ASD. The 3D TEE can be especially useful in characterizing the degree of rim deficiency. Additionally, the absence of aortic rim in the 0° modified 5-chamber view, termed a bald aorta, is especially high-risk for erosion, because the atrial free wall is directly fused to the aorta in this recess of the transverse sinus, and the relative expansion of the aorta during the cardiac cycle may result in device contact. Aortoatrial fistulas have also been rarely reported in this location.

Despite the higher risk of erosion, device closure with absent aortic rims is not a contraindication for device closure and can have comparable successful clinical outcomes. A recent study of a single center's experience in ASD closures found that the likelihood of procedural success, defined as device deployment without major complication, is significantly lower when there are multiple versus single deficient rims (86% vs 98%, vs 100% with sufficient rims).[31] Most unsuccessful deployments were due to technical or anatomic difficulty in deploying a device in stable position or a large ASD unsuitable for device closure. There was 1 occurrence (among 474 attempted closures) of device erosion and tamponade in a patient with absent aortic rim and a malaligned septum that occurred 3 days postimplantation, requiring emergent surgical repair. However, among those with devices successfully deployed, there was no difference in intermediate-term clinical outcomes (followed for a mean of 25 months) in cardiovascular events among the different rim morphologies.

Inconsistent posterior rim, best visualized in the basal SAX view, results in imprecise sizing that confers excess risk of perforation. The waist of the device is sturdy and can push on the posterior rim after deployment. The larger LA disc wedges between the aorta anteriorly and the LA free wall posteriorly, resulting in atrial trauma and erosion over time due to the motion of atrial contractions. This can be seen on the intraprocedural TEE as deformation of the aortic root by the device or tenting of the posterior free wall.

Other echocardiographic features are less consistently associated with erosion but should also be noted for closer follow-up (see Box 2). Septal malalignment in which the IAS favors 1 side of the aortic cusp rather than the midline tilts 1 of the device discs into the aorta. Dynamic ASDs are at increased risk due to difficulty of device sizing, as well as exaggerated movement of the atrial wall against the device. Oversizing the device by more than 1.5 times the ASD size, splaying of the discs around the aorta, and excessive movement of the deployed device were all found to be associated with erosion. Avoidance of oversizing has resulted in a substantial reduction in the rate of erosion. Whether splaying of the discs around the aorta should be avoided is a matter of controversy because some operators believe that the rigid ends of the discs jutting into the aorta may itself heighten the risk of erosion.[32] However, there is a consensus that oversizing should be avoided if possible and, if balloon sizing is used, the stop-flow method (previously described) should be used rather than using the diameter of the balloon waist when the defect is overstretched. Cardioform Septal Occluder device might be preferred for closure of smaller ASDs with deficient aortic rims, because this device is not associated with this complication. Erosions through the atrial free wall may be gradual and subacute in presentation. Therefore, even trace pericardial effusion on procedural or follow-up imaging warrants careful monitoring with serial imaging over the first day and week.

Postprocedure Follow-up Imaging

Based on these findings, a US Food and Drug Administration panel recommended frequent serial imaging by TTE in the first year postprocedure: at discharge, 1 week for Amplatzer devices, 1 month, 6 months, and 1 year after device implantation.[2,28] Follow-up studies should assess device positioning and stability, presence and degree of any residual shunt, any evidence of deformation or impingement on surrounding structures, presence and size of pericardial effusion and whether there is suggestion of device erosion, and presence of device thrombus. Over time with successful ASD closure, RV size and PASP may improve and normalize.

SUMMARY

ASD and PFOs are common congenital conditions diagnosed in adulthood. With improved device and imaging technology, percutaneous device closure of ASD and PFOs has become the preferred therapy when anatomically suitable. This article discussed the use of TTE, TEE, and ICE for diagnosis, preprocedural planning, intraprocedural guidance and monitoring, and postprocedural follow-up of percutaneous

ASD and PFO device closures. Advances in real-time 3D imaging complement and parallel evolving device technologies to make possible safer and more effective structural interventions.

REFERENCES

1. Schneider B, Zienkiewicz T, Jansen V, et al. Diagnosis of patent foramen ovale by transesophageal echocardiography and correlation with autopsy findings. Am J Cardiol 1996;77(14):1202–9.
2. Silvestry FE, Cohen MS, Armsby LB, et al. Guidelines for the echocardiographic assessment of atrial septal defect and patent foramen ovale: from the American Society of Echocardiography and Society for Cardiac Angiography and Interventions. J Am Soc Echocardiogr 2015;28(8):910–58.
3. Hagen PT, Scholz DG, Edwards WD. Incidence and size of patent foramen ovale during the first 10 decades of life: an autopsy study of 965 normal hearts. Mayo Clin Proc 1984;59(1):17–20.
4. Agmon Y, Khandheria BK, Meissner I, et al. Frequency of atrial septal aneurysms in patients with cerebral ischemic events. Circulation 1999;99(15):1942–4.
5. Tobis J, Shenoda M. Percutaneous treatment of patent foramen ovale and atrial septal defects. J Am Coll Cardiol 2012;60(18):1722–32.
6. Warnes CA, Williams RG, Bashore TM, et al. ACC/AHA 2008 guidelines for the management of adults with congenital heart disease: a report of the American College of Cardiology/American Heart Association Task Force on Practice Guidelines (Writing Committee to Develop Guidelines on the Management of Adults With Congenital Heart Disease). Developed in Collaboration With the American Society of Echocardiography, Heart Rhythm Society, International Society for Adult Congenital Heart Disease, Society for Cardiovascular Angiography and Interventions, and Society of Thoracic Surgeons. J Am Coll Cardiol 2008;52(23):e143–263.
7. Marriott K, Manins V, Forshaw A, et al. Detection of right-to-left atrial communication using agitated saline contrast imaging: experience with 1162 patients and recommendations for echocardiography. J Am Soc Echocardiogr 2013;26(1):96–102.
8. Nishimura RA, Tajik AJ. The Valsalva maneuver-3 centuries later. Mayo Clin Proc 2004;79(4):577–8.
9. McKenzie JA, Edwards WD, Hagler DJ. Anatomy of the patent foramen ovale for the interventionalist. Catheter Cardiovasc Interv 2009;73(6):821–6.
10. Carroll JD, Saver JL, Thaler DE, et al. Closure of patent foramen ovale versus medical therapy after cryptogenic stroke. N Engl J Med 2013;368(12):1092–100.
11. St. Jude Medical. AMPLATZER™ PFO Occluder for the prevention of recurrent ischemic stroke:

Sponsor's executive summary. Paper presented at: the U.S. Food and Drug Administration Circulatory System Devices Panel Meeting. Gaithersburg, May 24, 2015.
12. Hahn RT, Abraham T, Adams MS, et al. Guidelines for performing a comprehensive transesophageal echocardiographic examination: recommendations from the American Society of Echocardiography and the Society of Cardiovascular Anesthesiologists. J Am Soc Echocardiogr 2013;26(9):921–64.
13. Lang RM, Badano LP, Tsang W, et al. EAE/ASE recommendations for image acquisition and display using three-dimensional echocardiography. J Am Soc Echocardiogr 2012;25(1):3–46.
14. Simpson J, Lopez L, Acar P, et al. Three-dimensional echocardiography in congenital heart disease: an expert consensus document from the European Association of Cardiovascular Imaging and the American Society of Echocardiography. J Am Soc Echocardiogr 2017;30(1):1–27.
15. Kadakia MB, Silvestry FE, Herrmann HC. Intracardiac echocardiography-guided transcatheter aortic valve replacement. Catheter Cardiovasc Interv 2015;85(3):497–501.
16. Dhoble A, Nakamura M, Makar M, et al. 3D intracardiac echocardiography during TAVR without endotracheal intubation. JACC Cardiovasc Imaging 2016;9(8):1014–5.
17. Yared K, Baggish AL, Solis J, et al. Echocardiographic assessment of percutaneous patent foramen ovale and atrial septal defect closure complications. Circ Cardiovasc Imaging 2009;2(2):141–9.
18. Ponnuthurai FA, van Gaal WJ, Burchell A, et al. Safety and feasibility of day case patent foramen ovale (PFO) closure facilitated by intracardiac echocardiography. Int J Cardiol 2009;131(3):438–40.
19. Newton JD, Mitchell AR, Wilson N, et al. Intracardiac echocardiography for patent foramen ovale closure: justification of routine use. JACC Cardiovasc Interv 2009;2(4):369 [author reply: 369–70].
20. Rigatelli G, Pedon L, Zecchel R, et al. Long-term outcomes and complications of intracardiac echocardiography-assisted patent foramen ovale closure in 1,000 consecutive patients. J Interv Cardiol 2016;29(5):530–8.
21. Matsumura K, Gevorgyan R, Mangels D, et al. Comparison of residual shunt rates in five devices used to treat patent foramen ovale. Catheter Cardiovasc Interv 2014;84(3):455–63.
22. Amin Z, Hijazi ZM, Bass JL, et al. PFO closure complications from the AGA registry. Catheter Cardiovasc Interv 2008;72(1):74–9.
23. Krumsdorf U, Ostermayer S, Billinger K, et al. Incidence and clinical course of thrombus formation on atrial septal defect and patent foramen ovale closure devices in 1,000 consecutive patients. J Am Coll Cardiol 2004;43(2):302–9.

24. Abaci A, Unlu S, Alsancak Y, et al. Short and long term complications of device closure of atrial septal defect and patent foramen ovale: meta-analysis of 28,142 patients from 203 studies. Catheter Cardiovasc Interv 2013;82(7):1123–38.

25. Amin Z. Echocardiographic predictors of cardiac erosion after Amplatzer septal occluder placement. Catheter Cardiovasc Interv 2014;83(1):84–92.

26. Amin Z, Hijazi ZM, Bass JL, et al. Erosion of Amplatzer septal occluder device after closure of secundum atrial septal defects: review of registry of complications and recommendations to minimize future risk. Catheter Cardiovasc Interv 2004;63(4): 496–502.

27. DiBardino DJ, McElhinney DB, Kaza AK, et al. Analysis of the US Food and Drug Administration Manufacturer and User Facility Device Experience database for adverse events involving Amplatzer septal occluder devices and comparison with the Society of Thoracic Surgery congenital cardiac surgery database. J Thorac Cardiovasc Surg 2009; 137(6):1334–41.

28. Moore J, Hegde S, El-Said H, et al. Transcatheter device closure of atrial septal defects: a safety review. JACC Cardiovasc Interv 2013;6(5):433–42.

29. Divekar A, Gaamangwe T, Shaikh N, et al. Cardiac perforation after device closure of atrial septal defects with the Amplatzer septal occluder. J Am Coll Cardiol 2005;45(8):1213–8.

30. Podnar T, Martanovic P, Gavora P, et al. Morphological variations of secundum-type atrial septal defects: feasibility for percutaneous closure using Amplatzer septal occluders. Catheter Cardiovasc Interv 2001;53(3):386–91.

31. Kijima Y, Akagi T, Takaya Y, et al. Deficient surrounding rims in patients undergoing transcatheter atrial septal defect closure. J Am Soc Echocardiogr 2016;29(8):768–76.

32. Carroll JD. Device erosion. Catheter Cardiovasc Interv 2009;73(7):931–2.

Current Dataset for Patent Foramen Ovale Closure in Cryptogenic Stroke
Randomized Clinical Trials and Observational Studies

Olufunso W. Odunukan, MBBS, MPH*,
Matthew J. Price, MD

KEYWORDS

- Patent foramen ovale • Cryptogenic stroke • Paradoxic embolism

---

KEY POINTS

- Approximately one-third of all strokes are cryptogenic strokes and are associated with a patent foramen ovale (PFO) in up to 60% of all cases.
- The presumed biologic mechanisms of ischemic stroke in the setting of a PFO are paradoxic embolism through the interatrial shunt or embolism from in situ thrombosis.
- Several randomized clinical trials have been performed and late 6-year follow-up from one trial demonstrated superiority of device closure over standard-of-care medical therapy.

INTRODUCTION

Strokes can be catastrophic with devastating consequences, especially in the young and middle aged. Each year, approximately 795,000 people experience a new or recurrent stroke; 10% of these occur in people 18 to 50 years of age.[1] Thirty percent to 40% of ischemic strokes do not have an identified cause and are referred to as cryptogenic.[2,3] The statistical association between cryptogenic stroke and the presence of a patent foramen ovale (PFO) has long been established.[4] Although a PFO can be demonstrated in approximately 20% to 25% of the general population, it is much more frequent in patients who have suffered a cryptogenic stroke. In a series of contemporary experiences, the prevalence of PFO in cryptogenic stroke ranged from 21% to 63%.[4–6] Paradoxic embolism from the venous system or from thrombus formed in

situ has been presumed to be the causal mechanisms for this association.[7,8]

STUDIES OF THE EFFICACY OF MEDICAL THERAPY

The PFO in Cryptogenic Stroke Study (PICSS) was a 42-center cohort study that evaluated transesophageal echocardiographic findings in 630 stroke patients (265 with cryptogenic stroke and 203 with PFO) randomized to warfarin or aspirin. The goal of this study was to define the rate of recurrent stroke or death in stroke patients with or without PFO. There was no difference in the rate of recurrent ischemic stroke or death at 2-year follow-up in patients with or without a PFO in the overall population (14.8% vs 15.4%; hazard ratio [HR] 0.84; 95% confidence interval [CI]: 0.62, 1.48; $P = .84$) or in the cryptogenic stroke subgroup

---

Division of Cardiovascular Diseases, Scripps Clinic, 9898 Genesee Avenue, La Jolla, CA 92037, USA
* Corresponding author. Division of Cardiovascular Diseases, Scripps Clinic, Prebys Cardiovascular Institute, 9898 Genesee Avenue, Suite AMP-200, La Jolla, CA 92037.
E-mail address: Odunukan.olufunso@scrippshealth.org

Intervent Cardiol Clin 6 (2017) 525–538
http://dx.doi.org/10.1016/j.iccl.2017.05.007
2211-7458/17/© 2017 Elsevier Inc. All rights reserved.

(14.3% vs 12.7%; HR 1.17; 95% CI: 0.60, 2.37; P = .65). There was no significant difference in the risk of recurrence in patients with PFO randomized to warfarin or aspirin (16.5% vs 13.2%, HR 1.29; 95% CI: 0.63, 2.64, P = .49), although the study was underpowered to answer that question in this subgroup. The PICSS study established that medical therapy with warfarin or aspirin reduced the risk of recurrence of strokes in PFO patients to the same as those with identifiable causes.[2] This finding was corroborated in a meta-analysis of 15 observational studies involving 2548 patients with previous cryptogenic stroke or transient ischemic attack (TIA) managed medically, which showed that relative risk of recurrent neurologic events was similar in patients with and without PFO.[9] Using 4 of the 15 studies that had control groups (1081 patients), the pooled absolute rate of recurrent stroke or TIA was estimated at 4.0 events per 100 patient-years (PY) (95% CI: 3.5, 5.1), whereas the pooled absolute rate of recurrent stroke was estimated at 1.6 events per 100 PY. There was considerable heterogeneity in the estimates of the absolute rate of recurrent neurologic events for patients treated medically mainly due to major differences in how the diagnoses of cryptogenic stroke and PFO were reached as well as the determination of recurrent events. The choice of antiplatelet or anticoagulation in most studies was at the discretion of managing providers. Another meta-analysis of observational studies reported an annual incidence rate of 2.53 events (95% CI, 1.91–3.35) per 100 person-years among patients receiving medical therapy.[10]

The findings of observational studies evaluating the relative efficacy of antiplatelet and anticoagulation therapy for stroke reduction in PFO patients with cryptogenic stroke have generally been inconclusive.[11–14] The Targeted Antithrombotic Therapy in Cryptogenic Stroke with PFO study was a meta-analysis conducted to specifically answer this question.[15] The investigators pooled individual participant data of 2385 cryptogenic stroke patients with PFO treated medically (804 with anticoagulation and 1581 with antiplatelet therapy) from 12 databases, including the 3 randomized controlled trials comparing medical therapy with PFO closure. There was no significant difference in the primary composite outcome of recurrent stroke, TIA, or death (adjusted HR 0.76; 95% CI: 0.52, 1.12) or the secondary outcome of stroke alone (adjusted HR 0.75; 95% CI: 0.44, 1.27) in the patients managed with anticoagulation compared

with antiplatelet therapy. Although there was no significant heterogeneity of treatment effects in this meta-analysis, there were significant differences between treatment groups that might have led to confounding despite statistical adjustment.

In sum, studies of the natural history and of the medical therapy for cryptogenic stroke in PFO patients demonstrate fairly low yearly event rates (approximately 2.5 events per 100 PY), although this must be interpreted in the context of a relatively young patient population. Furthermore, there is a lack of robust data addressing whether anticoagulation or antiplatelet therapy is the preferred management strategy for prevention of stroke recurrence. The 2014 Guidelines for the Prevention of Stroke in Patients with Stroke and Transient Ischemic Attack recommend antiplatelet therapy in patients with an ischemic stroke or TIA and a PFO who are not undergoing anticoagulation therapy (Class I; Level of Evidence B); for patients with an ischemic stroke or TIA and both a PFO and a venous source of embolism, anticoagulation is indicated, depending on stroke characteristics (Class I; Level of Evidence A).[16]

OBSERVATIONAL STUDIES OF PERCUTANEOUS PATENT FORAMEN OVALE CLOSURE

Percutaneous PFO closure with an occluder device to reduce the risk of recurrent stroke was first described in 1992 in a study of 36 patients with right-to-left atrial shunting and presumed paradoxic emboli who were successfully implanted with the Bard Clamshell double-umbrella device (C. R. Bard Inc, Murray Hill, NJ) with minimal procedural morbidity.[17] A nonrandomized comparison of 308 cryptogenic stroke patients and PFO who underwent percutaneous closure with those that received medical treatment alone suggested that PFO closure may be especially beneficial in patients who have had more than one event in the past (Fig. 1) and may represent the highest-risk group.[12] It was noted in that study that events rates between PFO closure and medical therapy groups seemed to separate after 2 years of follow-up (Fig. 2), a finding attributed to possible noncompliance in patients treated medically. The benefit of closure may be attenuated in patients with incomplete PFO closure because residual shunting may make them prone to recurrent events in the immediate months following closure despite antithrombotic therapy because

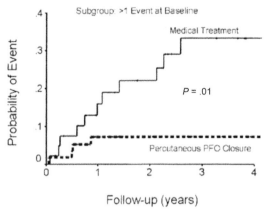

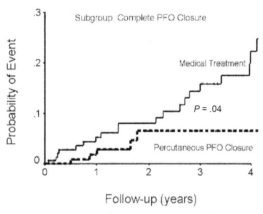

Follow-up (years)

Fig. 1. Comparison of time to recurrent stroke or TIA curves of patients with PFO closure versus medical therapy in the subgroup with more than 1 recurrent event. (*Adapted from* Windecker S, Wahl A, Nedeltchev K, et al. Comparison of medical treatment with percutaneous closure of patent foramen ovale in patients with cryptogenic stroke. J Am Coll Cardiol 2004;44(4):750–8.)

the device only becomes fully protective after complete endothelialization has occurred (Fig. 3).

Using Bayes' theorem, a meta-analysis designed to estimate the probability that a PFO in a patient with cryptogenic stroke was incidental concluded after evaluating 23 case control studies of the prevalence of PFO in patients with cryptogenic strokes compared with those with strokes of identifiable causes, that the probability was lower in patients greater

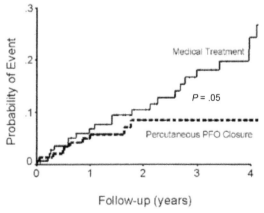

Follow-up (years)

Fig. 2. Kaplan-Meier curves of death, recurrent stroke, or TIA for PFO closure versus medical treatment. (*Adapted from* Windecker S, Wahl A, Nedeltchev K, et al. Comparison of medical treatment with percutaneous closure of patent foramen ovale in patients with cryptogenic stroke. J Am Coll Cardiol 2004;44(4):750–8.)

Fig. 3. Comparison of time to recurrent stroke or TIA curves in the subgroup with complete PFO closure. (*Adapted from* Windecker S, Wahl A, Nedeltchev K, et al. Comparison of medical treatment with percutaneous closure of patent foramen ovale in patients with cryptogenic stroke. J Am Coll Cardiol 2004;44(4):750–8.)

than 55 years old at 20% (95% CI: 16%, 25%) compared with 48% in older patients (95% CI: 34%, 66%). This probability was even much lower when a septal aneurysm was present.[18] Thus, these factors may play a role in the selection of PFO patients with cryptogenic strokes who are at high risk for recurrence of cerebrovascular events.[19]

Several observational studies have demonstrated the safety of percutaneous PFO closure with procedural success as high as 99%.[11,20–23] Among 352 patients who underwent percutaneous PFO closure with the Amplatzer Septal Occluder Device (St Jude Medical, Maple Grove, MN) (348, 98.9%) or the CardioSEAL occluder (NMT Medical Inc, Boston, MA) (4, 1.1%), the procedural complication rate was 3.4% and the rate of stroke or stroke and TIA was 0.9% and 2.8% at 1 and 4 years, respectively.[11] Some have proposed performing PFO closure with fluoroscopic guidance alone, without intracardiac echocardiographic guidance, with resultant shorter procedural times.[21]

OBSERVATIONAL STUDIES COMPARING DEVICE CLOSURE WITH MEDICAL THERAPY

Although many observational studies have studied recurrence rates of neurologic events in PFO patients with cryptogenic strokes after percutaneous device closure, very few of them had control arms of similar patients treated medically. To compound this problem, recurrent events without very long-term follow-up are rare in this patient population. Several attempts have therefore been made to adjust for these differences with meta-analyses and propensity studies.

Meta-analyses

In a meta-analysis of 39 observational studies involving 8185 patients treated with percutaneous PFO closure using several different devices (5 most prevalent: Amplatzer, Cardio-SEAL, PFOStar [Cardia Inc, Burnsville, MN], Star-flex, and Helex) and 19 studies involving 2142 patients managed with antiplatelet and/or anti-coagulant therapy,[14,24] the pooled incidence of recurrent neurologic events (stroke or TIA) was 0.78 per 100 PY (95% CI: 0.48–1.05 events per 100 PY) in patients treated with PFO closure compared with 4.39 events per 100 PY (95% CI: 3.20–5.59 events per 100 PY) in patients treated with medical management. Among the 10 studies involving 1886 patients that directly compared PFO closure with medical therapy, there was a significant 75% relative risk (RR: 0.25 [95% CI: 0.11, 0.58]) in the rate of recurrent stroke or TIA among patients who underwent percutaneous closure (Fig. 4). After adjustment for mean age, proportion of men in the study, and proportion of patients with atrial septal aneurysm, there was a significant reduction in recurrence by 3.5 events per 100 PY (95% CI:

2.1, 5.0; $P<.0001$) in patients treated with percutaneous closure compared with those treated with medical management.[14] The composite complication rate per 100 PY was estimated at 4.1 (95% CI: 3.2, 5.0) in the percutaneous closure group compared with 0.4 events (95% CI: 0, 0.9) in the medical management arm. Atrial arrhythmias were the most frequent complication after percutaneous closure, occurring in 3.9% (95% CI: 2.7, 6.1), and were most commonly associated with CardioSEAL (10.2/100 PY) and Starflex devices (9.0/100 PY) and least with the Amplatzer and the Helex devices. Device-related thrombosis occurred in 0.6% (95% CI: 0.3–0.9), most commonly with the Starflex device (NMT Medical Inc, Boston, MA). The rate of bleeding complications in the percutaneous closure arm was 1.7% (95% CI: 1.1, 2.4) in contrast to a rate of 1.1% (95% CI: 0, 2.5) in the medical therapy arm.

Propensity-Matched Analyses

In a prospective cohort study of 308 consecutive patients with cryptogenic stroke and PFO (150 PFO closure and 158 medical therapy) with a maximum follow-up of 15 years, a propensity score-matched analysis of 103 pairs of patients demonstrated better clinical outcomes associated with PFO closure compared with medical therapy. Patients were treated with 6 different devices

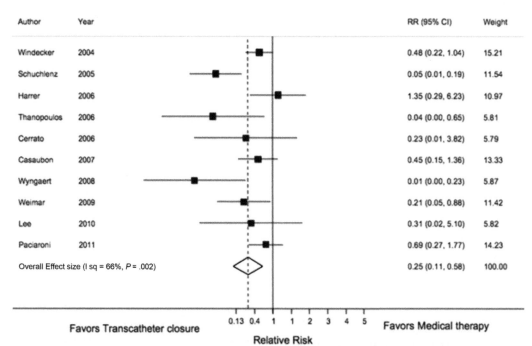

Fig. 4. Forest plot depicting a comparison of the risk of recurrent neurologic events in the transcatheter PFO closure group and medical management group in comparative studies. RR, relative risk. (*Adapted from* Agarwal S, Bajaj NS, Kumbhani DJ, et al. Meta-analysis of transcatheter closure versus medical therapy for patent foramen ovale in prevention of recurrent neurological events after presumed paradoxical embolism. JACC Cardiovasc Interv 2012;5(7):777–89.)

(Amplatzer PFO 36%, PFO STAR 28%, Sideris Buttoned (Custom Medical devices, Amarillo, TX) 16.7%, Angel Wing (Microvena Corporation, White Bear Lake, MN) 6.7%, Amplatzer ASD 6%, and CardioSEAL 5.3%.) Medically managed patients were treated with warfarin or antiplatelet therapy (aspirin or clopidogrel). The rate of recurrent stroke, TIA, or peripheral embolism was significantly lower with device closure compared with anticoagulant or antiplatelet therapy (11% vs 22%, HR 0.47, 95% CI: 0.20–0.94, $P = .033$).[19] This treatment effect was mostly related to a reduction in the recurrence of TIA. Although this observational study had the longest follow-up duration and attempted to minimize confounding by indication using propensity score matching, the variation in the devices used as well as the use of now obsolete devices constitute noteworthy limitations. In addition, the study included index events that may not have been related to PFO, particularly TIA without imaging evidence of an ischemic event. Moreover, some of the follow-up events may have been due to identifiable causes unrelated to the presence of a PFO.

In contrast, a recent propensity score–based analysis of similar endpoints in the Italian Project on Stroke in Young Adults registry showed no significant difference in the recurrence of a composite of stroke, TIA, or peripheral arterial embolism among 521 cryptogenic stroke patients aged 18 to 45 with a PFO followed from 2000 to 2012. Most devices used were Amplatzer occluders (86.8%), whereas CardioSEAL (1.9%), STARFlex (2.4%), Helex (2.4%), BioSTAR (NMT Medical Inc, Boston, MA) (1.9%), Premere (St Jude Medical, Maple Grove, MN) (3.3%), Figulla ASD occluder (Occlutech GmbH, Jena, Germany) (0.9%), and ATRIASEPT (Cardia Inc, Eagan, MN) (0.4%) comprised the remainder. At a median follow-up of 32 months in the device group and 36 months in the medical group, event rates were 7.3% and 10.5% (crude HR 0.72, 95% CI: 0.39–1.32, $P = .285$), respectively, and there was no significant difference in the propensity score adjusted outcomes (HR 0.69, 95% CI: 0.37–1.31). However, there seemed to be greater benefit to PFO closure in young patients aged less than 37 years (HR 0.19, 95% CI: 0.04–0.81, $P = .026$) and those with substantial right-to-left shunt (HR 0.19, 95% CI: 0.05–0.68, $P = .011$).[25]

RANDOMIZED CLINICAL TRIALS

Interpretation of the observational studies of medical versus invasive management of cryptogenic stroke and PFO is challenging given their conflicting results and substantial inherent bias.

Several randomized clinical trials have since explored the safety and efficacy of transcatheter PFO closure compared with medical therapy in patients with cryptogenic stroke.

CLOSURE I

CLOSURE I (Evaluation of the STARFlex Septal Closure System in Patients with a Stroke and/or Transient Ischemic Attack due to Presumed Paradoxical Embolism through a Patent Foramen Ovale) was a multicenter, randomized, open-label, 2-arm study that was designed to demonstrate superiority of the STARFlex device over medical therapy for the prevention of recurrent stroke or TIA in patients aged 18 to 60 years with cryptogenic stroke or TIA with a PFO. The trial planned to enroll 1600 patients, which would have provided 80% power to detect an expected treatment effect of the closure device of 50% assuming a 2-year stroke or TIA recurrence rate of 6% and 7% patient dropout. However, enrollment was slow, and the statistical plan was revised to decrease the sample size to 800 patients on the basis of an expected treatment effect of 66%. After an interim analysis indicated that this sample size would provide insufficient power, the trial ultimately enrolled only 909 patients, 72% of whom had an index cryptogenic stroke and 28% of whom had an index TIA. Patients allocated to device closure received dual antiplatelet therapy with aspirin and clopidogrel for 6 months and then maintenance-dose aspirin for 2 years. Patients allocated to medical therapy were treated with aspirin 325 mg daily and/or warfarin with a target international normalized ratio of 2.0 to 3.0 according to operator preference.[26] In the closure group, 405 of the 447 patients underwent attempted implantation of the device with an 89.4% success rate. At 2-year follow-up, there was no significant difference in the rate of the primary endpoint (5.5% in the closure group vs 6.8% in the medical therapy group, adjusted HR 0.78; 95% CI: 0.45, 1.35; $P = .37$) (Fig. 5). There were no significant differences in the 2-year rates of stroke (2.9% vs 3.1% in the closure group vs medical therapy group, respectively, adjusted HR 0.90, 95% CI: 0.41–1.98) or TIA (3.1% vs 4.1%, adjusted HR 0.75, 95% CI: 0.36–1.55). Patients allocated to device closure had an increased risk of atrial fibrillation (5.7% vs 0.7%, $P<.001$). There was no interaction between the presence of atrial septal aneurysm or the degree of shunting and the treatment effect of PFO closure. Two of the 12 strokes in the closure group were associated with device-related thrombus. A large proportion of the

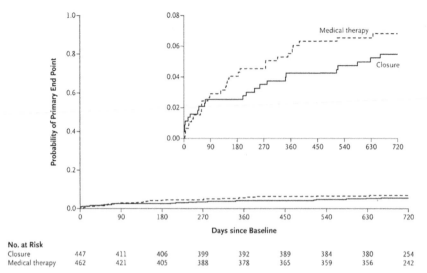

Fig. 5. Kaplan-Meier curves for the primary endpoint of stroke or TIA through 2 years of follow-up in the CLOSURE I trial. (*Adapted from* Furlan AJ, Reisman M, Massaro J, et al. Closure or medical therapy for cryptogenic stroke with patent foramen ovale. N Engl J Med 2012;366(11):991–9.)

recurrent neurologic events were due to identifiable causes. In addition to an overly optimistic anticipated treatment effect, significant limitations of this trial include the inclusion of TIA as criteria for enrollment and the commercial availability of PFO closure in an off-label fashion, which may have resulted in a study population less likely to benefit from PFO closure. In addition, effective closure with the device used in this trial was achieved in only 86% of patients at 6-month and 2-year follow-up.

PC TRIAL

The Clinical Trial Comparing Percutaneous Closure of Patent Foramen Ovale Using the Amplatzer PFO Occluder with Medical Treatment in Patients with Cryptogenic Embolism (PC Trial) was a multicenter study that enrolled 414 patients less than 60 years of age who had a documented PFO and imaging-verified cryptogenic stroke, TIA, or extracranial peripheral thromboembolic event. Patients were randomly assigned to either PFO closure with the Amplatzer PFO Occluder (St Jude Medical, Maple Grove, MN) or medical therapy with antiplatelet therapy or anticoagulation.[27] Device-treated patients received dual antiplatelet platelet therapy for up to 6 months. The enrolled sample size was estimated to provide 90% power to detect a reduction in the primary composite endpoint of death, nonfatal stroke, TIA, or peripheral embolism from 3% to ≤1% per year over a mean follow-up of 4.5 years. Implantation was attempted in 196 of the 204 patients in the closure group with a success rate of 95.9%. At a mean

follow-up of 4 years, transcatheter PFO did not significantly reduce the risk of the primary endpoint compared with medical therapy (cumulative incidence of 3.4% in the closure group vs 5.2% in the medical therapy group, HR 0.63; 95% CI: 0.24, 1.62; P = .34) (Fig. 6). Strokes were infrequent and numerically lower in the device arm, but this difference did not reach statistical significance (0.5% vs 2.4%, HR, 0.20; 95% CI, 0.02–1.72; P = .14). There was no difference in the rates of TIA between study arms (2.5% vs 3.3%, HR, 0.71; 95% CI, 0.23–2.24; P = .56). Unlike in the CLOSURE trial, PFO closure in the PC trial with the Amplatzer closure device was not associated with a statistically significant increase in atrial fibrillation compared with medical therapy, and there was no occurrence of device-associated thrombi.

Because the event rate of 5.2% in the medical therapy group was much less than the anticipated rate of 12% (3% per year), the study was considerably underpowered to detect the anticipated 66% reduction in relative risk in the closure group. Moreover, the inclusion of overall death as well as TIA in the primary endpoint may have diminished the ability of the trial to detect a treatment effect with PFO closure.

RESPECT TRIAL

The Randomized Evaluation of Recurrent Stroke Comparing PFO Closure to Established Current Standard of Care Treatment (RESPECT) was a multicenter, open-label clinical trial that was designed to demonstrate the superiority of

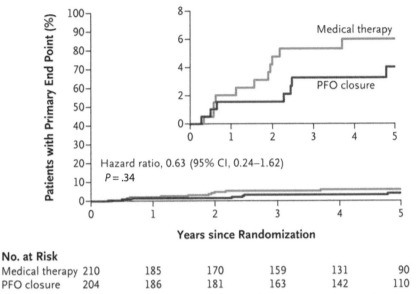

No. at Risk

Medical therapy 210	185	170	159	131	90
PFO closure 204	186	181	163	142	110

Fig. 6. Kaplan-Meier curves for the primary endpoint of death, nonfatal stroke, TIA, or peripheral embolism at 4-year follow-up in the PC trial. (*Adapted from* Meier B, Kalesan B, Mattle HP, et al. Percutaneous closure of patent foramen ovale in cryptogenic embolism. N Engl J Med 2013;368(12):1083–91.)

percutaneous PFO closure and medical therapy over medical therapy alone to prevent stroke recurrence in patients with imaging-confirmed cryptogenic stroke and PFO. A total of 1000 patients aged between 18 and 60 years were planned to be enrolled, which would provide 80% power to detect a 75% risk reduction in the primary composite endpoint of recurrent nonfatal ischemic stroke, fatal ischemic stroke, or early death after randomization, assuming 2-year event rates of 4.3% in the medical therapy group and 1.05% in the closure group at α of 0.05. As the event rates were expected to be low, the study was to be stopped after the first 25 observed events. The trial ultimately enrolled 980 patients who were randomly assigned to transcatheter closure with the Amplatzer PFO Occluder or medical therapy alone (any of aspirin, warfarin, clopidogrel, and aspirin combined with extended-release dipyridamole).[28] Patients who were randomized to device therapy were treated with antiplatelet therapy after the procedure (81–325 mg of aspirin plus clopidogrel for a month followed by aspirin monotherapy for 5 months). Among the patients randomized to medical management, 25% were treated with warfarin and the remainder with antiplatelet agents. In the closure group, 464 (93%) underwent implantation with technical and procedural success rates of 99.1% and 96.1%, respectively. There was relatively more attrition in the medical therapy compared with

the closure group (dropout rate 17% vs 9.2%), resulting in a significant difference in the duration of follow-up between the 2 groups (1184 patient-years vs 1375 patient-years, P = .009). The initial analysis occurred after 25 primary events. At this juncture, according to intention-to-treat, PFO closure led to a 51% risk reduction in recurrent events, which did not reach statistical significance (0.66 events per 100 PY in the closure group compared with 1.38 events per 100 PY in the medical therapy group, HR 0.49; 95% CI: 0.22, 1.11; P = .08). Notably, 3 of the 9 primary events in the closure group occurred in individuals who did not have a device implanted at the time of recurrence. There was a statistically significant reduction the rate of the primary endpoint with device closure according to the prespecified per-protocol analysis (0.46 vs 1.30 events per 100 PY [HR, 0.37; 95% CI: 0.14, 0.96; P = .03]) and the as-treated analysis (0.39 vs 1.45 events per 100 PY [HR, 0.27; 95% CI: 0.10, 0.75; P = .007]). In addition, prespecified subgroup analyses suggested that closure may be particularly beneficial in patients with concomitant atrial septal aneurysm and those with substantial shunts.

Serious adverse events were infrequent. Rates of atrial fibrillation did not differ significantly between the closure and medical therapy groups (3.0% vs 1.5%, P = .13). However, there was greater incidence of deep venous thrombosis and pulmonary embolism in the closure group

(1.2%) compared with 0.2% in the medical therapy group (P = .12). Although speculative, this may be due to relative differences in antithrombotic therapy between the randomized groups in these patients with possibly greater thrombogenic potential.

The relative benefit of PFO closure may increase over time, because the absolute yearly risk of ischemic events may be relatively low, but these young patients are continuously exposed to an ongoing hazard of ischemic events over time. Therefore, continued follow-up of trials of PFO closure may demonstrate significant benefit over time. Recently, the final, 6-year follow-up of RESPECT trial was reported (Dr David Thaler, unpublished data, 2017).

At a mean follow-up of 5.9 years (6.3 years or 3141 PY in the device group, and 5.5 years or 2669 PY in the medical management group), PFO closure led to a statistically significant reduction in the risk of recurrent ischemic stroke according to intention-to-treat analysis (**Fig. 7**). Specifically, there were 18 strokes in the group randomly assigned to device closure compared with 28 strokes in the group assigned to medical management (HR 0.55, 95% CI: 0.305, 0.999, P = .046). Because patients had aged considerably during the course

of follow-up (with more than 10 years of follow-up in some patients), the treatment effect of PFO closure was diluted by the occurrence of ischemic strokes with an identified cause in both study arms. The magnitude of effect was even larger for the prevention of recurrent cryptogenic stroke. For this endpoint, PFO closure led to a statistically significant 62% risk reduction (HR 0.38, 95% CI: 0.18, 0.79, P = .007) (**Fig. 8**). Similarly, in patients censored at 60 years of age, there were 12 ischemic strokes in the PFO occluder group compared with 25 in the medical therapy group, resulting in a significant 58% risk reduction (HR 0.42, 95% CI: 0.21, 0.83, P = .100) (**Fig. 9**). Subgroup analyses were consistent with the initial findings that patients with substantial shunt size and those with atrial septal aneurysm derived particular benefit from PFO closure.

An important limitation of the RESPECT trial is the presence of retention bias resulting from the larger dropout rate in the medical therapy group, presumably due in part to preference for available off-label PFO closure with non–US Food and Drug Administration (FDA) -approved devices. In addition, high-risk patients may have been treated with off-label PFO closure outside the trial with consequent entry bias.

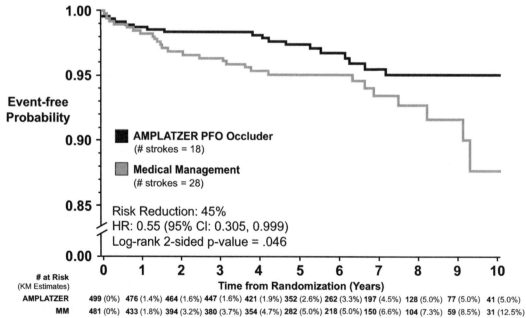

Fig. 7. Kaplan-Meier curves among the PFO closure arm and the medical therapy arm in the intention-to-treat population for the primary endpoint of recurrent ischemic stroke. (*Courtesy of* David Thaler. Long-term study results show that PFO closure is more effective than medical management in preventing recurrent stroke. Presented at the Transcatheter Cardiovascular Therapeutics (TCT) Scientific Sessions. Washington, DC, November 1, 2016; with permission.)

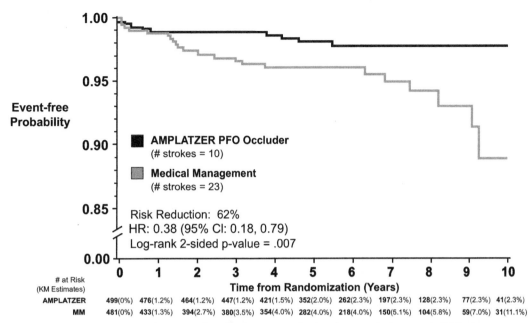

Fig. 8. Long-term recurrent ischemic stroke of unknown mechanism-free survival curves in PFO closure group versus medical management in the final intention-to-treat analysis of the RESPECT trial. (*Courtesy of* David Thaler. Long-term study results show that PFO closure is more effective than medical management in preventing recurrent stroke. Presented at the Transcatheter Cardiovascular Therapeutics (TCT) Scientific Sessions. Washington, DC, November 1, 2016; with permission.)

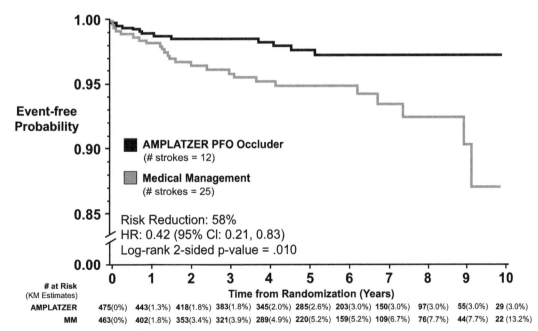

Fig. 9. Long-term recurrent ischemic stroke–free survival curves in patients censored at age 60 in the final intention-to-treat analysis of the RESPECT trial. (*Courtesy of* David Thaler. Long-term study results show that PFO closure is more effective than medical management in preventing recurrent stroke. Presented at the Transcatheter Cardiovascular Therapeutics (TCT) Scientific Sessions. Washington, DC, November 1, 2016; with permission.)

When interpreting the results of the RESPECT trial in the context of the CLOSURE and PC trials, it becomes apparent that although all 3 clinical trials set out to test the superiority of PFO closure, critical factors such as entry criteria, the choice of device, estimation of incidence rates of the outcome, and thus, sample size determination, the selection of primary end points, and follow-up duration all played a role in the relative ability of each of the trials to detect the effect of PFO closure on prevention of recurrent cryptogenic strokes. RESPECT, with its strict entry criteria, mechanistically reasonable endpoints, adequate power, and the longest follow-up duration, had the most robust design and demonstrated a benefit for PFO closure.

META-ANALYSIS OF CLINICAL TRIALS

Given that none of the 3 randomized trials met their primary endpoint by intention-to-treat (although RESPECT did meet its endpoint after long-term follow-up), meta-analyses may further clarify the treatment effect of PFO closure on the recurrence of neurologic events in cryptogenic strokes compared with medical therapy and may help to identify particular subgroups who may derive particular benefit.[28] A plethora of such meta-analyses were conducted with conflicting results before the long-term follow-up from RESPECT was concluded. Those results were unsurprising because direct comparisons of the 3 randomized studies may likely be error prone given the different efficacy and safety profiles of the StarFlex device used in Closure I and the Amplatzer PFO occluder in the RESPECT and PC trials.[29]

A pooled analysis of the individual patient data included the 2303 subjects in the 3 randomized controlled trials, followed for a total of 5849 person-years with 108 composite endpoint events. There was a lower but nonsignificant difference in the unadjusted risk of the primary composite outcome of stroke, TIA, or death in patients receiving PFO closure compared with medical therapy (HR 0.69; 95% CI: 0.47, 1.091; $P = .053$), and a significant reduction in the risk of the primary outcome following covariate adjustment for known predictors of stroke recurrence or PFO-related mechanisms in the RoPE score (HR: 0.68; 95% CI: 0.46–1.00; $P = .049$). PFO closure reduced the rate of ischemic stroke in both unadjusted and adjusted analyses (HR: 0.58; 95% CI: 0.34–0.98; $P = .043$; and HR: 0.58; 95% CI: 0.34–0.99; $P = .044$, respectively).

In an analysis limited to the 2 studies (PC and RESPECT) using the Amplatzer PFO Occluder (1394 patients; 54 events), the findings were consistent with the overall analysis, although the point estimates were slightly lower, particularly for the endpoint of ischemic stroke (unadjusted HR, 0.39; 95% CI: 0.19, 0.82; $P = .013$).[30] There was no significant heterogeneity demonstrated. The study also confirmed the relatively low absolute yearly rates of recurrent stroke in patients less than 60 years of age regardless of the mode of management with an event rate of 0.98 strokes and 1.8 composite events per 100 person-years across both groups, although these may become substantial in absolute terms over the long term in these young individuals. The investigators speculate that overestimation of the event rates in the planning phase may have resulted in inadequate power of the individual studies to detect a difference between study arms. In addition, the consistent signal of benefit of PFO closure for prevention of recurrent ischemic stroke suggests that this endpoint is a more reliable outcome with regard to treatment effect of PFO closure compared with TIA and overall mortality, which may be influenced by mechanisms other than the presence of a PFO.

A network meta-analysis of 4 randomized trials[26–28,31] with 2963 patients and 9309 PY suggested that the success of the PFO closure for secondary prevention of cryptogenic strokes depended on which of the devices used. The Amplatzer PFO occluder had the highest probability of efficacy at 77.1% compared with 20.9% for the Helex, 1.7% with StarFlex, and 0.4% with medical therapy.[32] Similarly, device type appeared to influence the rates of specific adverse effects: compared with medical treatment, the risk of new onset atrial fibrillation was highest with the StarFlex (7.6%), whereas the risk was lower with the Amplatzer PFO Occluder (2.14%) and the Helex Septal Occluder (W.L. Gore & Co, Flagstaff, AZ) (1.33%). Similarly, another meta-analysis of 3311 patients in 4 randomized trials and 17 observational studies specifically compared long-term efficacy and safety of PFO closure with each of the 2 antithrombotic strategies. The study identified a significant net clinical benefit of percutaneous PFO closure (odds ratio [OR] 0.30; 95% CI: 0.18, 0.51; $P<.00001$) compared with antiplatelet therapy with an absolute excess risk of 1.7% per year for stroke or TIA for antiplatelet therapy. In addition, there was a significant net clinical benefit of PFO closure when compared with anticoagulation (OR 0.32; 95% CI: 0.18,

0.59; $P = .003$) with an absolute excess risk of 2.1% per year for major bleeding with anticoagulation.[33]

With the overall low event rates, it is likely that the short follow-up in the randomized studies (CLOSURE I 2 years, RESPECT 2.6 years, and PC 4.1 years) may have been inadequate to detect a treatment effect.[34] Longer-term follow-up of these patients as was done in RESPECT is therefore critical. Furthermore, CLOSURE I was limited by difficulty in patient recruitment (909/1600) as well as inclusion of outcome events with identifiable causes.[35] The RESPECT and PC trials were also hampered by slow recruitment, considerable attrition, small event rates, and enrollment after the period of highest risk.[36] It must be emphasized that patient enrollment may have been hindered by the off-label treatment of high-risk patients with PFO closure outside of the randomized clinical trials with resultant entry and retention bias.[19,28,34]

COST-EFFECTIVENESS

A cost analysis by Picket and colleagues[37] attributed higher expenditures to PFO closure related to procedural costs with a cost of $16,213 per patient. They projected that PFO closure became cost-effective (<$50,000 per quality life-year gained) at 2.6 years and the mean cost of PFO closure per patient is exceeded by that of medical treatment at the 30-year mark. They concluded that reduced event rates together with the long-term costs of medical treatment may eventually offset the initial high costs in patients with PFO closure via the transcatheter approach.

RISK OF PARADOXICAL EMBOLISM DATABASE AND SCORE

Because the overall yearly recurrence rates of cryptogenic strokes are fairly low, and in many patients, the PFO may be an innocent bystander, stratifying the PFO-attributable risk of recurrent events is critical. The Risk of Paradoxical Embolism (RoPE) study was a global collaboration that created the largest collection of cryptogenic stroke patients with known PFO with adjudicated events.[5] These data describe the natural history of these patients and guide decision-making regarding diagnosis and secondary prevention of cryptogenic strokes.

Kent and colleagues[7] devised the RoPE score as an index to predict the probability of a concurrent PFO in a patient with cryptogenic stroke. This score is derived from a set of simple clinical variables: younger age, presence of cortical stroke on neuroimaging, and absence of vascular risk factors (hypertension, diabetes mellitus, smoking, and previous stroke). Thus, superficial strokes in the youngest patients without vascular risk factors generate the highest score. The 10-point RoPE score also stratifies patients by the probability that a PFO when present is stroke-related or merely incidental, that is, it can be used to attempt to quantify the risk attributable to a PFO for a particular patient with a cryptogenic stroke. The absolute yearly recurrence rate of stroke is relatively low in the high RoPE score strata (ie, those with the highest PFO-attributable risk), whereas the absolute recurrence rate is highest in patients with multiple risk factors for ischemic stroke. For example, in patients with a RoPE score of 9 to 10, where the PFO prevalence was 73% (95% CI: 66%–79%), the 2-year recurrence rate was 2% (95% CI: 0%–4%) compared with a 20% recurrence rate (95% CI: 12%–28%) in the lowest 0 to 3 stratum with PFO prevalence of 23% (95% CI: 19%–26%). Appropriate risk stratification has considerable implications as randomized clinical trials comparing PFO closure with medical therapy may have had inadequate sample sizes based on inaccurate assumptions of the recurrence rates of PFO-attributable strokes.[7] Although the absolute yearly risk may be low in patients with high RoPE scores, the lifetime risk in these younger patients is substantial. Given the low yearly rate of recurrence, longer follow-up is likely required to detect a significant risk reduction with any intervention. The combination of the clinical variables in the RoPE score with specific high-risk PFO characteristics, such as large shunt size, spontaneous shunting at rest, or concomitant atrial septal aneurysm, may help to identify individuals at higher risk of recurrence who may derive the greatest benefit from PFO closure. Other predictors of PFO-associated cryptogenic strokes may include a history of deep vein thrombosis or pulmonary embolism, migraine, recent prolonged travel, Valsalva at onset of event, or stroke upon awakening.[38]

CURRENT STATE OF US FOOD AND DRUG ADMINISTRATION APPROVAL

The FDA approved the Amplatzer PFO occluder in October 2016 with the indication for the "percutaneous transcatheter closure of a PFO to reduce the risk of recurrent ischemic stroke in patients, predominantly between the ages of 18 and 60 years, who have had a cryptogenic stroke due to presumed paradoxical embolism, as determined by a neurologist and cardiologist following an evaluation to exclude known causes of ischemic stroke." A multidisciplinary approach is therefore critical to the management of cryptogenic strokes, including close collaboration between neurology and cardiology.

FUTURE DIRECTIONS

Pending observational studies and randomized clinical trials will provide further clarity regarding the safety and efficacy of percutaneous PFO closure to prevent recurrent stroke. The PFO Access Registry is assessing the effect of PFO closure with the Amplatzer PFO occluder in patients with ≥2 cryptogenic strokes due to presumed paradoxic embolism through the PFO while on medical therapy.[39] The GORE Helex Septal Occluder/GORE Cardioform Septal Occluder and Antiplatelet Medical Management for Reduction of Recurrent Stroke or Imaging-Confirmed TIA in Patients With Patent Foramen Ovale (REDUCE) randomized clinical trial (clinicaltrials.gov identifier NCT00738894) aims to evaluate the safety and efficacy of PFO closure with the GORE Helex or Cardioform Septal Occluders compared with medical management with antiplatelet therapy to reduce the risk of recurrent stroke or TIA in patients with a history of cryptogenic stroke or imaging-confirmed TIA.[40] The results of the REDUCE trial, which could lead to FDA approval of the Cardioform device for PFO closure, are due to be reported in late 2017. It remains to be seen whether the FDA will approve this device if it is demonstrated to be safe, but the overall trial shows no clinical benefit due to being underpowered to show a difference in clinical endpoints; the regulatory outcome of such a scenario will certainly affect the ability of novel devices to gain regulatory approval short of large-scale efficacy trials. Future randomized trials to evaluate the clinical efficacy of transcatheter closure compared with medical therapy will require novel designs to address the problems of entry and retention bias prevalent in the previous randomized clinical trials. Furthermore, the optimal antithrombotic therapy in patients with cryptogenic stroke and PFO remains unknown. Comparative randomized clinical trials of various antithrombotic regimens including those in individuals undergoing PFO closure are necessary. Novel oral anticoagulants are currently been studied in the cryptogenic stroke population.[41,42]

SUMMARY

Although transcatheter PFO closure for cryptogenic stroke has been in use for more than 2 decades, indications and patient selection have remained controversial. Collaborative, observational studies have provided insight into risk-stratification to identify patients in whom PFO closure may provide the greatest potential. Long-term follow-up from randomized clinical studies has provided clarity regarding the efficacy of PFO closure in secondary stroke prevention.

REFERENCES

1. Writing Group Members, Mozaffarian D, Benjamin EJ, Go AS, et al. Heart disease and stroke statistics-2016 update: a report from the American Heart Association. Circulation 2016;133(4):e38–360.
2. Homma S, Sacco RL, Di Tullio MR, et al. Effect of medical treatment in stroke patients with patent foramen ovale: patent foramen ovale in Cryptogenic Stroke Study. Circulation 2002;105(22):2625–31.
3. Yaghi S, Elkind MS. Cryptogenic stroke: a diagnostic challenge. Neurol Clin Pract 2014;4(5): 386–93.
4. Lechat P, Mas JL, Lascault G, et al. Prevalence of patent foramen ovale in patients with stroke. N Engl J Med 1988;318(18):1148–52.
5. Thaler DE, Di Angelantonio E, Di Tullio MR, et al. The risk of paradoxical embolism (RoPE) study: initial description of the completed database. Int J Stroke 2013;8(8):612–9.
6. Senadim S, Bozkurt D, Çabalar M, et al. The role of patent foramen ovale in cryptogenic stroke. Noro Psikiyatr Ars 2016;53(1):60–3.
7. Kent DM, Ruthazer R, Weimar C, et al. An index to identify stroke-related vs incidental patent foramen ovale in cryptogenic stroke. Neurology 2013;81(7): 619–25.
8. Windecker S, Meier B. Is closure recommended for patent foramen ovale and cryptogenic stroke? Patent foramen ovale and cryptogenic stroke: to close or not to close? Closure: what else! Circulation 2008;118(19):1989–98.
9. Almekhlafi MA, Wilton SB, Rabi DM, et al. Recurrent cerebral ischemia in medically treated patent foramen ovale: a meta-analysis. Neurology 2009; 73(2):89–97.
10. Kitsios GD, Dahabreh IJ, Abu Dabrh AM, et al. Patent foramen ovale closure and medical treatments for secondary stroke prevention: a systematic review of observational and randomized evidence. Stroke 2012;43(2):422–31.
11. Ford MA, Reeder GS, Lennon RJ, et al. Percutaneous device closure of patent foramen ovale in

patients with presumed cryptogenic stroke or transient ischemic attack: the Mayo Clinic experience. JACC Cardiovasc Interv 2009;2(5):404–11.'

12. Windecker S, Wahl A, Nedeltchev K, et al. Comparison of medical treatment with percutaneous closure of patent foramen ovale in patients with cryptogenic stroke. J Am Coll Cardiol 2004;44(4):750–8.

13. Stern S, Cohen MJ, Gilon D, et al. Cryptogenic stroke in a patient with a PFO: a decision analysis. Am J Med Sci 2008;335(6):457–64.

14. Agarwal S, Bajaj NS, Kumbhani DJ, et al. Meta-analysis of transcatheter closure versus medical therapy for patent foramen ovale in prevention of recurrent neurological events after presumed paradoxical embolism. JACC Cardiovasc Interv 2012; 5(7):777–89.

15. Kent DM, Dahabreh IJ, Ruthazer R, et al. Anticoagulant vs. antiplatelet therapy in patients with cryptogenic stroke and patent foramen ovale: an individual participant data meta-analysis. Eur Heart J 2015;36(35):2381–9.

16. Kernan WN, Ovbiagele B, Black HR, et al. Guidelines for the prevention of stroke in patients with stroke and transient ischemic attack: a guideline for healthcare professionals from the American Heart Association/American Stroke Association. Stroke 2014;45(7):2160–236.

17. Bridges ND, Hellenbrand W, Latson L, et al. Transcatheter closure of patent foramen ovale after presumed paradoxical embolism. Circulation 1992; 86(6):1902–8.

18. Alsheikh-Ali AA, Thaler DE, Kent DM. Patent foramen ovale in cryptogenic stroke: incidental or pathogenic? Stroke 2009;40(7):2349–55.

19. Wahl A, Jüni P, Mono ML, et al. Long-term propensity score-matched comparison of percutaneous closure of patent foramen ovale with medical treatment after paradoxical embolism. Circulation 2012; 125(6):803–12.

20. Stanczak LJ, Bertog SC, Wunderlich N, et al. PFO closure with the Premere PFO closure device: acute results and follow-up of 263 patients. EuroIntervention 2012;8(3):345–51.

21. Siddiqui IF, Michaels AD. Percutaneous patent foramen ovale closure using Helex and Amplatzer devices without intraprocedural echocardiographic guidance. J Interv Cardiol 2011;24(3):271–7.

22. Mirzaali M, Dooley M, Wynne D, et al. Patent foramen ovale closure following cryptogenic stroke or transient ischaemic attack: long-term follow-up of 301 cases. Catheter Cardiovasc Interv 2015;86(6): 1078–84.

23. Moon J, Kang WC, Kim S, et al. Comparison of outcomes after device closure and medication alone in patients with patent foramen ovale and cryptogenic stroke in Korean population. Yonsei Med J 2016;57(3):621–5.

24. Freund MA, Reeder GS, Cabalka AK, et al. Percutaneous device closure of patent foramen ovale for cryptogenic strokes/transient ischemic attacks. JACC Cardiovasc Interv 2012;5(11):1189 [author reply: 1189].

25. Pezzini A, Grassi M, Lodigiani C, et al. Propensity score-based analysis of percutaneous closure versus medical therapy in patients with cryptogenic stroke and patent foramen ovale: the IPSYS registry (Italian Project on Stroke in Young Adults). Circ Cardiovasc Interv 2016;9(9) [pii:e003470].

26. Furlan AJ, Reisman M, Massaro J, et al. Closure or medical therapy for cryptogenic stroke with patent foramen ovale. N Engl J Med 2012;366(11):991–9.

27. Meier B, Kalesan B, Mattle HP, et al. Percutaneous closure of patent foramen ovale in cryptogenic embolism. N Engl J Med 2013;368(12):1083–91.

28. Carroll JD, Saver JL, Thaler DE, et al. Closure of patent foramen ovale versus medical therapy after cryptogenic stroke. N Engl J Med 2013;368(12):1092–100.

29. Rohrhoff N, Vavalle JP, Halim S, et al. Current status of percutaneous PFO closure. Curr Cardiol Rep 2014;16(5):477.

30. Kent DM, Dahabreh IJ, Ruthazer R, et al. Device closure of patent foramen ovale after stroke: pooled analysis of completed randomized trials. J Am Coll Cardiol 2016;67(8):907–17.

31. Hornung M, Bertog SC, Franke J, et al. Long-term results of a randomized trial comparing three different devices for percutaneous closure of a patent foramen ovale. Eur Heart J 2013;34(43):3362–9.

32. Stortecky S, da Costa BR, Mattle HP, et al. Percutaneous closure of patent foramen ovale in patients with cryptogenic embolism: a network meta-analysis. Eur Heart J 2015;36(2):120–8.

33. Patti G, Pelliccia F, Gaudio C, et al. Meta-analysis of net long-term benefit of different therapeutic strategies in patients with cryptogenic stroke and patent foramen ovale. Am J Cardiol 2015;115(6): 837–43.

34. Riaz IB, Dhoble A, Mizyed A, et al. Transcatheter patent foramen ovale closure versus medical therapy for cryptogenic stroke: a meta-analysis of randomized clinical trials. BMC Cardiovasc Disord 2013;13:116.

35. Hernandez J, Moreno R. Percutaneous closure of patent foramen ovale: "closed" door after the last randomized trials? World J Cardiol 2014;6(1):1–3.

36. Sharma M. ACP Journal Club. Patent foramen ovale closure and medical therapy did not differ for recurrence after cryptogenic stroke. Ann Intern Med 2013;159(4):JC4.

37. Pickett CA, Villines TC, Ferguson MA, et al. Cost effectiveness of percutaneous closure versus medical therapy for cryptogenic stroke in patients with a patent foramen ovale. Am J Cardiol 2014;114(10): 1584–9.

38. Ozdemir AO, Tamayo A, Munoz C, et al. Crypto-genic stroke and patent foramen ovale: clinical clues to paradoxical embolism. J Neurol Sci 2008; 275(1–2):121–7.

39. PFO ACCESS Registry. 2017. Available at: https://clinicaltrials.gov/show/NCT00583401. Accessed February 12, 2017.

40. GORE HELEX septal occluder/GORE septal occluder for patent foramen ovale (PFO) closure in stroke pa-tients - The Gore REDUCE Clinical Study (HLX 06–03). 2017. Available at: https://clinicaltrials.gov/show/NCT00738894. Accessed February 12, 2017.

41. RE-SPECT ESUS Dabigatran etexilate for sec-ondary stroke prevention in patients with embolic stroke of undetermined source. 2017. Available at: https://www.clinicaltrials.gov/ct2/show/NCT02239120. Accessed March 11, 2017.

42. NAVIGATE ESUS Rivaroxaban versus aspirin in secondary prevention of stroke and prevention of systemic embolism in patients with recent embolic stroke of undetermined source (ESUS). 2017. Available at: https://www.clinicaltrials.gov/ct2/show/NCT02313909. Accessed March 11, 2017.

Patent Foramen Ovale and Migraine Headache

David Hildick-Smith, MD, BM, BChir*, Timothy M. Williams, BA, BM, BCh

---

KEYWORDS

• Migraine • PFO • PFO closure • Migraine aura • Structural cardiology

---

KEY POINTS

- Migraine headache is a common and debilitating illness affecting a significant proportion of the population.
- The is an association of migraine headache and the presence of patent foramen ovale (PFO), with higher prevalence of migraine in patients with PFO and high prevalence of PFO in patients with migraine.
- Potential pathologic mechanisms include microemboli; fluctuations in vasoactive substances in the arterial circulation; and transient hypoxia, caused by right to left shunting in the circulation through a PFO.
- Percutaneous PFO closure has been reported to reduce the burden of migraine in patients with PFO; however, this reduction has failed to reach statistical significance in large, prospective trials.
- Further trials are warranted to explore whether a subset of patients with migraine with PFO would benefit from PFO closure.

INTRODUCTION

Migraine is a common disorder including migraine aura and debilitating migraine headaches occurring in episodes that often significantly affect patients' lives.[1,2] Symptoms typically consist of a unilateral headache, often pulsatile, and associated other complaints such as photophobia, nausea, phonophobia, and aura. There is much debate regarding the association of patent foramen ovale (PFO) with migraine, and therefore, much discussion about potential pathologic mechanisms and possible treatments, including percutaneous closure.

Percutaneous PFO closure was first performed in 1992[3] and since then has been used for treatment of paradoxic embolization in stroke, transient ischemic attack (TIA), decompression illness, peripheral embolization, and migraine. Despite this, the role for closure in migraine has not been clearly defined because of controversy over its efficacy. This article discusses the evidence for an association between PFO and migraine, possible pathologic mechanisms, and the evidence for percutaneous PFO closure as a treatment in patients with PFO and migraine.

MIGRAINE AND ITS ASSOCIATION WITH PATENT FORAMEN OVALE

Migraine is a common disease in the Western world, affecting around 12% of the population.[4] It is more common in women, with a male to female ratio of around 3:1, and has a peak of incidence in the middle age of life, with fewer affected in adolescence and after the age of 60 years.[1] Migraine carries a significant burden to those with the disease and significant numbers of patients miss work or school days because of the illness. One-quarter to one-third of patients have aura preceding, or during, their attacks of migraine headache. The aura can take a variety of forms of both positive and negative

---

Disclosure: D. Hildick-Smith has received advisory and consultancy fees from Gore, St Jude, and Occlutech.
Sussex Cardiac Centre, Brighton and Sussex University Hospitals, Eastern Road, Brighton, BN2 5BE, UK
* Corresponding author.
E-mail address: david.hildick-smith@bsuh.nhs.uk

neurologic symptoms. Most commonly these are visual but can cover a spectrum including sensory and motor symptoms. Typically, the aura of migraine was considered to occur before the onset of headache, but the two occur simultaneously for many migraineurs.[5]

The traditional hypothesis of migraine pathophysiology was that migraines occur because of changes in cerebral blood flow from vasodilatation and constriction; however, in recent years this has been rebuffed and the focus has turned to primary neuronal dysfunction as the underlying pathologic mechanism.[6,7]

Both the headache of migraine and the aura have been linked to a phenomenon known as cortical spreading depression.[6,8,9] Cortical spreading depression is a wave of cortical depolarization that both excites and depresses neurologic activity in its path. This phenomenon causes the aura of migraine,[10] in addition to the headache associated with classic migraine attacks. Migraine headache without aura is likely to be caused by cortical spreading depression in unconscious areas of the brain leading to headache but without conscious aura symptoms.[8]

Earlier studies suggested an increased incidence of migraine both with and without aura in patients with PFO, with a large study of patients who had cryptogenic stroke showing a significantly higher burden of migraine in patients with PFO compared with those without.[11] A cohort study in 1999 showed that the finding of a PFO, assessed by transcranial Doppler (TCD), was more common in patients with migraine with aura compared with controls.[12]

A systematic review in 2008 considered the association of PFO and migraine with a final analysis of 18 articles,[13] finding a significant association between migraine in patients with PFO, and also for the finding of PFO in patients with migraine. The association was present for both migraine with aura and migraine without aura. The findings of improved migraine symptoms in patients undergoing PFO closure in this study also supported a possible causal link between PFO and migraine. Another systematic review in 2013 also concluded that PFO and migraine were linked, and that the effect of closure was positive overall on migraine symptoms and continued to hint at a causal link.[14]

A more recent meta-analysis including 5572 patients across 21 studies was published in 2015.[15] Across all patients there was a significant association in the prevalence of migraine with aura and PFO relative to controls, with an odds ratio of 3.36 (95% confidence interval, 2.04–5.55). This association was also true for a group of patients who experienced migraine both with and without aura, but there was no significant association between patients with migraine who did not experience aura.

There are also studies showing a lack of association between PFO and migraine; however, none had the same level of evidence as a meta-analysis or systematic review. A cross-sectional study of 1101 elderly patients self-reporting symptoms of migraine failed to show a correlation between PFO and migraine,[16] with PFO assessed by transthoracic echocardiography and bubble contrast. Similarly, a case-control study with a total of 288 participants concluded that there was no increased PFO prevalence (assessed by transthoracic echocardiography and TCD) in migraineurs compared with controls.[17]

Potential explanations for differences in data include a variety of methods by which the presence of PFO is assessed, with different echocardiographic assessments between different data sets, and different thresholds at which a PFO is diagnosed.[18] There is a higher level of evidence from meta-analyses and systematic reviews to support an association between migraine with aura and the presence of a PFO than there is to refute it, but evidence of a causal link for PFO and migraine without aura is limited.

POTENTIAL PATHOLOGIC MECHANISMS OF PATENT FORAMEN OVALE AND MIGRAINE

Two main theories have been postulated to explain a causative link between PFO and migraine, the first of which is that right to left shunt across a PFO allows microemboli and metabolites from the venous circulation to enter the systemic circulation and cause cerebral irritation. In experimental models, hypoxemia has been shown as a potential trigger of cortical spreading depression,[9] and platelet activity and aggregation have been shown to be increased in patients who get migraines, particularly around the timing of acute attacks.[19] Furthermore, studies investigating the role of aspirin and oral anticoagulation in preventing migraine attacks have yielded positive results.[20,21] These findings point toward a potential mechanism of paradoxic microemboli and localized ischemia providing a migraine trigger (Fig. 1).

Metabolites such as serotonin crossing the PFO from venous to systemic circulation has also been suggested as a cause. Serotonin is released from aggregating platelets[19] as well

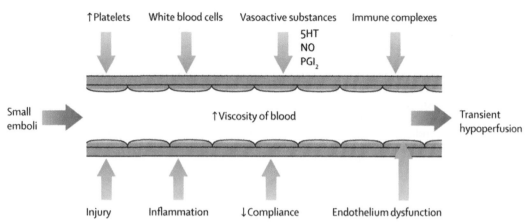

Fig. 1. Cerebral blood vessels are important for the triggering of cortical spreading depression and the pathophysiology of migraine aura. In patients with PFO, brief periods of local and mild hypoperfusion may develop as a consequence of microemboli arising from the venous circulation, or might develop in other conditions in response to injury to the vessel wall, local release of vasoactive substances, increased blood viscosity, circulating immune complexes, endothelial dysfunction, enhanced platelet-endothelial interaction, or platelet-leucocyte interaction, among other mechanisms. 5HT, serotonin; PGI_2, prostacyclin. (*Adapted from* Dalkara T, Nozari A, Moskowitz MA. Migraine aura pathophysiology: the role of blood vessels and microembolisation. Lancet Neurol 2010;9(3):309–17.)

as being present in venous blood, usually being deactivated in the lungs when no right to left shunt is present. In PFO, blood is potentially shunted away from the lungs and therefore active metabolites may not be deactivated in the usual way,[22] and arterial peaks of serotonin levels have been associated with triggering migraines.[23]

The second theory regarding PFO and migraine causation is that transient hypoxia caused by right to left shunting of blood may be the cause of migraine. Shunt across a PFO can occur during rest and stress, and in several other scenarios,[24] and this transient hypoxia may lead to the irritant trigger of migraine in some patients.[22]

The inherent problems with these theories are numerous,[25] and perhaps chief among them is that paradoxic embolization is a random event, whereas migraine tends to have a pattern that migraineurs experience on each occasion. Further studies are required in this area to clarify a pathologic connection between migraine and PFO.

EVIDENCE FOR PATENT FORAMEN OVALE CLOSURE

Early reports of PFO closure indicated a positive effect for percutaneous closure of PFO on migraine symptoms. Several observational, mostly retrospective, studies, in which the rationale for PFO closure was a paradoxic embolic event, showed that migraine symptoms were

improved among migraineurs following closure, with resolution of attacks in many cases.[26–30] There is evidence that in some cases PFO closure may trigger migraine symptoms,[31] although overall data from these early investigations suggest benefit.

A more recent prospective study of 80 patients with high-risk features for paradoxic embolism and high symptom burden showed a significant benefit with PFO closure at 2-year follow up, with complete resolution of migraine aura in 96.8% of the patients with aura, and improved symptoms in 87.5% of all patients with migraine regardless of the presence of aura.[32] A further prospective study of 305 patients undergoing PFO closure following a cerebrovascular event, of whom 77 patients were migraineurs, showed similarly good results from PFO closure with improvement in migraine symptoms in 89% of those patients over a median follow-up period of 28 months.[33]

Despite results from nonrandomized trials showing promise for PFO closure as a treatment of migraine, larger randomized trials have generally been less positive. A total of 3 major trials have been completed to date, with published results of 2 and the results of the third presented but not published.

The MIST (Migraine Intervention with STAR-Flex Technology) trial was the first randomized clinical trial to be undertaken.[34] This trial randomized 147 patients with frequent migraine with aura that was refractory to 2 preventive medications to either PFO closure with the

STARFlex device or a sham procedure. Patients were excluded if they had experienced a previous cerebrovascular accident. The trial was blinded to the patients and the investigators assessing the patients during follow-up. The primary end point was headache cessation. Follow-up at 6 months showed no benefit for PFO closure (4% headache-free response in both groups), and secondary end points were also not met. Post hoc analysis of the data showed 2 outliers in the implant group responsible for one-fifth of all headache days, and, when these patients were removed from analysis, there was a significant reduction in median total migraine headache days per month for the PFO closure group (37% vs 26% reduction, $P = .027$). Importantly, all patients were given dual antiplatelet therapy with aspirin and clopidogrel during the first 90 days, which may have contributed to some improvement in symptoms. There were

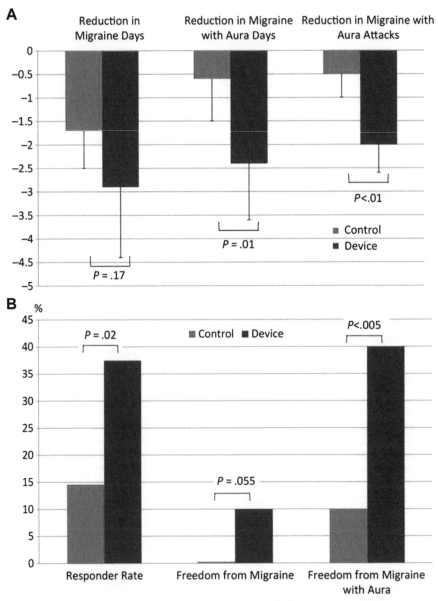

Fig. 2. PFO closure for migraine headache in the PRIMA randomized clinical trial. (A) Reduction in migraine days (primary end point) and reduction of migraine with aura days and migraine with aura attacks (bar graph with 95% confidence intervals). (B) Responder rate and number of patients free of migraine and free of migraine with aura. (Adapted from Mattle HP, Evers S, Hildick-Smith D, et al. Percutaneous closure of patent foramen ovale in migraine with aura, a randomized controlled trial. Eur Heart J 2016;37(26):2029–36.)

transient adverse effects in both arms of the trial but a higher number of serious adverse effects in the PFO closure group.

The PRIMA (Percutaneous Closure of Patent Foramen Ovale in Migraine with Aura) trial[35] was an open-label randomized trial of PFO closure with the AMPLATZER PFO Occluder (St Jude Medical, St Paul, MN) versus medical management in patients with migraine with aura and PFO. No sham procedure was included in the trial. The primary end point was a reduction in monthly migraine days 9 to 12 months after randomization compared with an average of 3 months before randomization. The trial was planned to enroll 144 patients but was halted early because of slow recruitment after 107 patients were enrolled. Medical therapy for both groups included aspirin for 6 months and clopidogrel for 3 months after randomization.

The primary end point, the reduction in migraine days per month, was reduced by 2.9 days in the closure group versus 1.7 days in the control arm, but this difference did not reach statistical significance ($P = .17$). In a post hoc analysis, PFO closure led to a significant reduction in the mean number of migraine with aura days per month compared with control (-2.4 vs -0.6 days, $P = .0141$). PFO closure also significantly reduced the number of migraine attacks with aura (-2.0 vs -0.5; $P = .0003$; **Fig. 2**). As in the MIST trial, there was a higher incidence of serious adverse events in the closure group, but all resolved during follow-up with no lasting effects.

The PREMIUM (Prospective, Randomized Investigation to Evaluate Incidence of Headache Reduction in Subjects with Migraine and PFO Using the AMPLATZER PFO Occluder to Medical Management) study is a double-blind, randomized, sham-controlled trial of PFO closure with the AMPLATZER PFO Occluder device as a treatment of migraine with and without aura in patients with PFO; the results have been presented but not yet published.[36] A total of 230 patients were enrolled who experienced migraine that was refractory to medical treatment, and were randomized to PFO closure or continued medical therapy. The primary end point, a 50% reduction in migraine attacks per month at 10 to 12 months after randomization, was not met, with 38% of the closure group reaching this target compared with 32% of the sham procedure group. Similarly to the PRIMA trial, there was a greater response to PFO closure in patients who had migraine with aura. In these patients, there was a response rate of 49% in the closure group compared with 23%

in the sham arm ($P = .015$). This enhanced effect was also true for cure of symptoms: among patients with aura, complete remission occurred in 10.8% of those undergoing PFO closure, compared with 1.5% in the control arm ($P = .02$). Only 1 adverse clinical event was reported at 12 months by the investigators.

The only meta-analysis of data for PFO closure as a treatment of migraine was published before the PRIMA trial, and therefore mainly includes retrospective studies for which PFO closure was performed following a stroke or TIA.[37] Data from MIST are included and the conclusions are generally positive, with suggestion of migraine cure in 46% of patients (95% confidence interval, 25%–67%).

Therefore, the evidence for the efficacy of PFO closure as a treatment of migraine in patients with PFO mainly originates from retrospective analyses of patients who underwent PFO closure for an indication other than migraine. The 3 randomized controlled trials (RCTs) completed to date did not reach their primary end points. However, there is strong suggestion from secondary analyses that there is a subgroup of patients for whom PFO closure is beneficial, particularly those patients who have migraine with aura. Clearly further trials are needed to answer fully the question of benefit in a prospective fashion.

SUMMARY

There is an association of increased migraine prevalence in patients with PFO, and an increased prevalence of PFO in patients with migraine, although the link between the two disorders and possible pathologic explanations are not fully elucidated. Early experience of PFO closure as a treatment of migraine in patients with PFO was positive, but unexpectedly negative results have been provided by RCTs investigating PFO closure prospectively. There seems to be a subset of patients, among migraineurs with aura, for whom PFO closure is likely to be beneficial, but further large trials are needed to support this proposition. Until these larger trials are completed, the evidence is inconclusive on the efficacy of PFO closure as a treatment of migraine, and it cannot be recommended for routine use.

REFERENCES

1. Lipton RB, Bigal ME, Diamond M, et al. Migraine prevalence, disease burden, and the need for preventive therapy. Neurology 2007;68(5):343–9.

2. Launer LJ, Terwindt GM, Ferrari MD. The prevalence and characteristics of migraine in a population-based cohort: the GEM study. Neurology 1999; 53(3):537–42. Available at: http://www.ncbi.nlm.nih. gov/pubmed/10449117. Accessed April 16, 2017.

3. Bridges ND, Hellenbrand W, Latson L, et al. Transcatheter closure of patent foramen ovale after presumed paradoxical embolism. Circulation 1992; 86(6):1902–8.

4. Lipton RB, Stewart WF, Diamond S, et al. Prevalence and burden of migraine in the United States: data from the American Migraine Study II. Headache 2001;41(7):646–57. Available at: http://www.ncbi. nlm.nih.gov/pubmed/11554952. Accessed April 16, 2017.

5. Hansen JM, Lipton RB, Dodick DW, et al. Migraine headache is present in the aura phase: a prospective study. Neurology 2012;79(20):2044–9.

6. Charles A. Advances in the basic and clinical science of migraine. Ann Neurol 2009;65(5):491–8.

7. Charles A. Vasodilation out of the picture as a cause of migraine headache. Lancet Neurol 2013; 12(5):419–20.

8. Takano T, Nedergaard M. Deciphering migraine. J Clin Invest 2009;119(1):16–9.

9. Lauritzen M. Pathophysiology of the migraine aura. The spreading depression theory. Brain 1994; 117(Pt 1):199–210. Available at: http://www.ncbi. nlm.nih.gov/pubmed/7908596. Accessed April 16, 2017.

10. Hadjikhani N, Sanchez Del Rio M, Wu O, et al. Mechanisms of migraine aura revealed by functional MRI in human visual cortex. Proc Natl Acad Sci U S A 2001;98(8):4687–92.

11. Lamy C, Giannesini C, Zuber M, et al. Clinical and imaging findings in cryptogenic stroke patients with and without patent foramen ovale: the PFO-ASA study. Atrial septal aneurysm. Stroke 2002;33(3): 706–11. Available at: http://www.ncbi.nlm.nih.gov/ pubmed/11872892. Accessed April 16, 2017.

12. Anzola GP, Magoni M, Guindani M, et al. Potential source of cerebral embolism in migraine with aura: a transcranial Doppler study. Neurology 1999;52(8): 1622–5. Available at: http://www.ncbi.nlm.nih.gov/ pubmed/10331688. Accessed April 16, 2017.

13. Schwedt T, Demaerschalk B, Dodick D. Patent foramen ovale and migraine: a quantitative systematic review. Cephalalgia 2008;28(5):531–40.

14. Lip PZ, Lip GY. Patent foramen ovale and migraine attacks: a systematic review. Am J Med 2014;127(5): 411–20.

15. Takagi H, Umemoto T. A meta-analysis of case-control studies of the association of migraine and patent foramen ovale. J Cardiol 2016;67(6): 493–503.

16. Rundek T, Elkind MS, Di Tullio MR, et al. Patent foramen ovale and migraine: a cross-sectional study from the Northern Manhattan Study (NOMAS). Circulation 2008;118(14):1419–24.

17. Garg P, Servoss SJ, Wu JC, et al. Lack of association between migraine headache and patent foramen ovale: results of a case-control study. Circulation 2010;121(12):1406–12.

18. Zito C, Dattilo G, Oreto G, et al. Patent foramen ovale: comparison among diagnostic strategies in cryptogenic stroke and migraine. Echocardiography 2009;26(5):495–503. Available at: http://www.ncbi. nlm.nih.gov/pubmed/19452605. Accessed April 16, 2017.

19. Borgdorff P, Tangelder GJ. Migraine: possible role of shear-induced platelet aggregation with serotonin release. Headache 2012;52(8):1298–318.

20. Buring JE, Peto R, Hennekens CH. Low-dose aspirin for migraine prophylaxis. JAMA 1990; 264(13):1711–3. Available at: http://www.ncbi.nlm. nih.gov/pubmed/2204739. Accessed April 16, 2017.

21. Rahimtoola H, Egberts AC, Buurma H, et al. Reduction in the intensity of abortive migraine drug use during coumarin therapy. Headache 2001;41(8): 768–73. Available at: http://www.ncbi.nlm.nih.gov/ pubmed/11576200. Accessed April 16, 2017.

22. Sharma A, Gheewala N, Silver P. Role of patent foramen ovale in migraine etiology and treatment: a review. Echocardiography 2011;28(8):913–7.

23. Schwedt TJ, Dodick DW. Patent foramen ovale and migraine–bringing closure to the subject. Headache 2006;46(4):663–71.

24. Naqvi TZ, Rafie R, Daneshvar S. Original investigations: potential faces of patent foramen ovale (PFO PFO). Echocardiography 2010;27(8):897–907.

25. Gupta VK. Patent foramen ovale closure and migraine: science and sensibility. Expert Rev Neurother 2010;10(9):1409–22.

26. Azarbal B, Tobis J, Suh W, et al. Association of interatrial shunts and migraine headaches: impact of transcatheter closure. J Am Coll Cardiol 2005; 45(4):489–92.

27. Schwerzmann M, Wiher S, Nedeltchev K, et al. Percutaneous closure of patent foramen ovale reduces the frequency of migraine attacks. Neurology 2004;62(8):1399–401. Available at: http://www.ncbi. nlm.nih.gov/pubmed/15111681. Accessed April 16, 2017.

28. Reisman M, Christofferson RD, Jesurum J, et al. Migraine headache relief after transcatheter closure of patent foramen ovale. J Am Coll Cardiol 2005;45(4):493–5.

29. Wahl A, Kunz M, Moschovitis A, et al. Long-term results after fluoroscopy-guided closure of patent foramen ovale for secondary prevention of paradoxical embolism. Heart 2008;94(3):336–41.

30. Wahl A, Praz F, Tai T, et al. Improvement of migraine headaches after percutaneous closure of

patent foramen ovale for secondary prevention of paradoxical embolism. Heart 2010;96(12):967–73.

31. Kato Y, Kobayashi T, Ishido H, et al. Migraine attacks after transcatheter closure of atrial septal defect. Cephalalgia 2013;33(15):1229–37.

32. Rigatelli G, Dell'avvocata F, Cardaioli P, et al. Improving migraine by means of primary transcatheter patent foramen ovale closure: long-term follow-up. Am J Cardiovasc Dis 2012;2(2):89–95. Available at: http://www.ncbi.nlm.nih.gov/pubmed/22720197. Accessed April 16, 2017.

33. Trabattoni D, Fabbiocchi F, Montorsi P, et al. Sustained long-term benefit of patent foramen ovale closure on migraine. Catheter Cardiovasc Interv 2011;77(4):570–4.

34. Dowson A, Mullen MJ, Peatfield R, et al. Migraine Intervention with STARFlex Technology (MIST) Trial: a prospective, multicenter, double-blind, sham-controlled trial to evaluate the effectiveness of patent foramen ovale closure with STARFlex septal repair implant to resolve refractory migraine headache. Circulation 2008;117(11):1397–404.

35. Mattle HP, Evers S, Hildick-Smith D, et al. Percutaneous closure of patent foramen ovale in migraine with aura, a randomized controlled trial. Eur Heart J 2016;37(26):2029–36.

36. Tobis J, Charles A, Silberstein SD, et al. TCT-30 PREMIUM Trial: double blind study of percutaneous closure of patent foramen ovale with the AMPLATZER® PFO Occluder as a treatment for migraine with or without aura. J Am Coll Cardiol 2015;66(15). http://dx.doi.org/10.1016/j.jacc.2015.08.076.

37. Butera G, Biondi-Zoccai GG, Carminati M, et al. Systematic review and meta-analysis of currently available clinical evidence on migraine and patent foramen ovale percutaneous closure: much ado about nothing? Catheter Cardiovasc Interv 2010;75(4):494–504.

Patent Foramen Ovale Closure for Hypoxemia

Jonathan M. Tobis, MD, FACC, MSCAI[a],*, Deepika Narasimha, MD[b],
Islam Abudayyeh, MD[b]

KEYWORDS

- Patent foramen ovale • Hypoxemia • Right-to-left shunting • COPD • Platypnea-orthodeoxia

KEY POINTS

- Hypoxemia may occur in the presence of a patent foramen ovale (PFO) caused by right-to-left shunt across the interatrial septum.
- Right-to-left shunting can be exacerbated by clinical conditions that alter the relative pressure between the right and left atria (eg, obstructive sleep apnea, chronic obstructive pulmonary disease, and pulmonary hypertension) or by changes in the anatomic relationship between the inferior vena cava and the foramen ovale caused by surgery or other conditions that may cause cardiac rotation.
- A PFO is one cause of platypnea-orthodeoxia (dyspnea and hypoxemia while upright, which improves in the recumbent position), in addition to liver and lung disease.
- PFO closure may successfully treat hypoxemia in selected cases.

INTRODUCTION

Several clinical syndromes are associated with patent foramen ovale (PFO), including stroke caused by paradoxic embolism, migraine headaches with aura, and decompression sickness. Although the link between these disorders and PFO has been studied extensively, the associations between hypoxemia-related conditions such as chronic obstructive pulmonary disease (COPD), obstructive sleep apnea (OSA), and the platypnea-orthodeoxia syndrome (POS) are not fully defined. Case reports linking PFO to hypoxemia that is out of proportion to the severity of lung disease have been described over the last 2 decades.[1–3] This article describes the mechanisms linking hypoxemia with the presence of a PFO, the clinical conditions in which PFO may play a role in contributing to hypoxemia, and the role of PFO closure in management.

PATENT FORAMEN OVALE AND HYPOXEMIA

In the fetal circulation, blood from the inferior vena cava (IVC) flows from the right atrium (RA) into the left atrium (LA) through the foramen ovale, which acts as a one-way valve. This valve ensures that oxygenated blood from the placenta directly enters the systemic circulation, and bypasses the nonaerated, amniotic fluid–filled lungs. The remaining oxygenated blood that gets into the right ventricle (RV) is directed through the ductus arteriosus into the descending aorta, thus also bypassing the nonfunctional lungs. The IVC is aligned with the PFO by the eustachian valve, which facilitates the IVC flow directly across the septum. Blood from the superior vena cava (SVC) meanwhile is directed down into the RA and across the tricuspid valve (Fig. 1). After birth, the pulmonary vascular resistance decreases, leading to a decrease in RA

Disclosures: The authors state that no commercial or financial conflicts of interest or funding sources exist for this article.

[a] Division of Cardiology, Department of Medicine, David Geffen School of Medicine at UCLA, 10833 Le Conte Avenue, Factor Building CHS, Room B-976, Los Angeles, CA 90095, USA; [b] Division of Cardiology, Interventional Cardiology, Loma Linda University Health, 11234 Anderson Street, MC 2434, Loma Linda, CA 92354, USA
* Corresponding author.
E-mail address: jtobis@mednet.ucla.edu

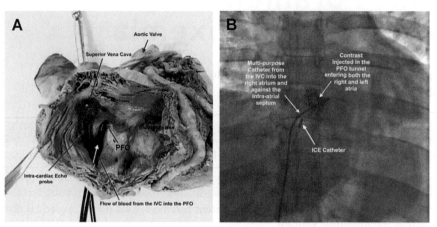

Fig. 1. (A) Gross anatomy showing the atrial septum from the right atrial side. The delivery catheter follows the course of the IVC and into the PFO. The SVC is angled away from the PFO and points toward the tricuspid valve. (B) Fluoroscopic image showing the course of a catheter as it enters the RA via the IVC and is directed toward the PFO. ICE, intracardiac echocardiography.

pressure. As the LA pressure exceeds the RA pressure, the septum primum closes against the septum secundum. With time, the septum primum and secundum fuse leaving behind the fossa ovalis. For approximately 20% of the population this fusion remains incomplete, resulting in a PFO.[4–6] In most people who have a PFO, it is an incidental finding and not associated with symptoms or hypoxemia. However, right-to-left shunting (RLS) of blood can occur during any activity that increases venous return and right atrial pressure, such as the release of the Valsalva maneuver. It is estimated that a cryptogenic stroke occurs in 1 in 1000 people per year who have a PFO. Of the patients with PFO who have some related symptom, only 3% present with symptomatic hypoxemia.

Although RLS causing hypoxemia is rare in patients without increased right-sided pressures, there have been reports of significant hypoxemia in patients with normal right-sided pressures.[7] Godart and colleagues[7] report a series of 11 patients with PFO who presented with significant dyspnea and cyanosis, which subsided after percutaneous closure of the atrial defect. Six of the 11 patients also had POS, in which the hypoxemia occurs on sitting or standing up. Various theories exist to explain RLS in patients with normal right-sided pressures. These theories include preferential blood flow streaming from the IVC to the LA because of the presence of a large eustachian valve.[8,9] Another theory describes the presence of a systolic right-to-left atrial pressure gradient in conditions such as RV infarction, right atrial myxoma, and mechanical ventilation.[10,11] In these cases, inspiration, the Valsalva maneuver, and changes in

posture exacerbate RLS. In the 11 patients described earlier, the investigators observed that all of the patients had rotated atrial septa toward the horizontal axis such that the PFO was more directly in line with the blood flow from the IVC. Note that this phenomenon has also been noted in patients with ascending aortic aneurysms that may distort the septum, or after pneumonectomy and abdominal surgery, which are thought to alter the anatomic orientation or opening height of the PFO. The incidence and degree of shunting also increase when the septum primum is aneurysmal or highly mobile (Fig. 2).[9,12]

Establishing that an RLS through a PFO is primarily responsible for hypoxemia or cyanosis in patients without increased right-sided pressures can be challenging. Persistent desaturations despite administration of 100% oxygen therapy should alert clinicians to the possibility of an RLS. A transesophageal echocardiogram (TEE) showing cross-septal flow on color Doppler or contrast administration can help confirm the diagnosis. In addition, on cardiac catheterization, there is a step-down in the oxygen saturation levels in the LA compared with the pulmonary veins, with return to normal blood saturation after occlusion of the PFO using a soft balloon sizing catheter.[7] Once identified, quantifying the degree of hypoxemia caused by RLS can be difficult. A low pulmonary vein oxygen saturation might indicate a mixed picture in which pulmonary disease is a contributor to hypoxemia, whereas a step-down of saturations in the LA compared with the pulmonary veins should indicate that an RLS through the PFO plays a larger role. Crossing the PFO to obtain

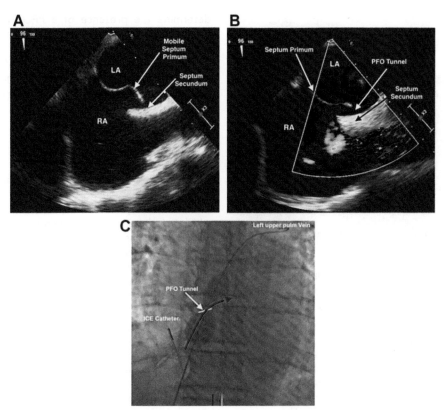

Fig. 2. (*A*) Large PFO with an aneurysmal septum primum. (*B*) Color-flow echocardiogram showing significant flow across PFO caused by a mobile septum primum. (*C*) Fluoroscopic image showing a sizing balloon in the PFO. The sizing balloon shows a wide-diameter (12 mm) PFO tunnel (*white line*). The red arrow indicates the shunt pathway if the balloon was not present.

saturation samples in the LA and pulmonary veins is usually straightforward and can be performed using a multipurpose catheter and a J-tipped guidewire. Once in the left atrium, it is important to be meticulous with catheter manipulation and aspiration so as to prevent clots or air from entering the LA (see **Fig. 2**; **Fig. 3**).

PATENT FORAMEN OVALE AND CHRONIC OBSTRUCTIVE PULMONARY DISEASE

Patients with COPD have been noted to have a higher prevalence of PFO. Soliman and colleagues[2] evaluated the prevalence of PFO in patients with severe COPD (forced expiratory volume in 1 second [FEV_1] <50%, and FEV_1/forced vital capacity ratio <50%) compared with control subjects without COPD by means of contrast TEE and cough or Valsalva maneuvers. The prevalence of PFO in patients with COPD was twice that of normal controls (70% vs 35%). In addition, the investigators also noted transient systemic arterial desaturations in half of these patients, the severity of which was

proportional to the degree of pulmonary hypertension. Note that the prevalence of PFO in this study was much higher compared with other population-based studies. The prevalence of diagnosing a PFO depends on the threshold used during the contrast study. Hacievliyagil and colleagues[13] similarly found a higher prevalence of PFO in patients with COPD (23 out of 52 compared with 10 out of 50 controls). The investigators used transthoracic echocardiography (TTE) with contrast at rest and with Valsalva to detect PFO. They also found that patients with COPD with PFO had lower oxygen saturations, shorter 6-minute walk test (6MWT) durations, and longer duration of disease compared with patients with COPD without PFO. In contrast, a study by Shaikh and colleagues[14] did not find a statistically significant increase in the prevalence of PFO in 50 patients with COPD compared with 50 controls (46% vs 30%; *P* = .15). The investigators did find that large shunts were more common in patients with COPD. They used both contrast TTE and transcranial Doppler (TCD) to make the diagnosis of PFO, with most shunts

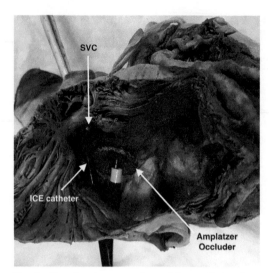

SVC

ICE catheter

Amplatzer
Occluder

Fig. 3. The direct access of a guiding catheter from the IVC into the PFO and deployment of an Amplatzer device within the septum.

being grade 2 or less (grade 0, up to 3 microbubbles; grade 1, 3–10; grade 2, 11–30; grade 3, 31–100; grade 4, >100; grade 5, microbubbles filling the spectrum for more than 3 cardiac cycles). Note that TCD is a more sensitive tool for the detection of PFO than TTE. The ultimate standard for diagnosing a PFO is to perform a right heart catheterization (RHC) and show that a guidewire can cross the atrial septum. With RHC as the standard, a TCD grade 3 or greater correlates to the presence of a PFO. TCD grades 1 or 2 are unlikely to be caused by a PFO and are ascribed to pulmonary passage of microbubbles.

Martolini and colleagues[15] evaluated patients enrolled in the Global Initiative for Chronic Obstructive Lung Disease (GOLD) stage II COPD study to assess the effects of PFO on arterial oxygen saturation and exercise tolerance, and whether the RLS through the PFO increased during exercise. Twenty-two patients were enrolled in the study, and contrast-enhanced TCD was used to diagnose PFO in these patients. A PFO was identified in 12 of the 22 patients (54%). Furthermore, although the prevalence of PFO was higher in this population than in the general population, patients with PFO did not have a decreased exercise tolerance or a reduced 6MWT duration compared with those without a PFO. Although there was an increase in RLS during exercise, there were no functional consequences from a PFO in this group of patients. The limitations of the study include a small sample size, very few large PFOs, and absence of a control group. In addition, inaccuracies may arise during TCD to

determine the presence of a PFO in patients with COPD, because TCD cannot accurately distinguish between intracardiac and intrapulmonary shunting, and patients with COPD can have significant intrapulmonary shunting. Differentiating between the two depends on timing of the bubbles and operator experience.

PATENT FORAMEN OVALE AND PULMONARY HYPERTENSION

Up to one-third of patients with COPD have associated pulmonary hypertension.[15–17] COPD is characterized by ventilation-perfusion mismatch, which results in blood flowing to capillaries supplying diseased or nonfunctional alveoli. This condition causes a progressive increase in pulmonary artery pressure (PAP) caused by hypoxia-induced pulmonary vasoconstriction.[18,19] An increase in PAP leads to an increase in RA pressure, which can lead to increased RLS in the presence of a PFO. Patients with COPD and PFO therefore can have an RLS as an additive cause for hypoxemia.

The phenomenon of clinical deterioration following shunt closure in patients with congenital heart disease and Eisenmenger syndrome is described in the early surgical literature.[20] This phenomenon led to the hypothesis that an RLS may be necessary to release the excessive PAP in patients with pulmonary hypertension. Austin and colleagues[21] showed improvement in systemic pressures and exercise tolerance with creation of an RLS via atrial septostomy in dogs with experimental RV hypertension. Similarly, in patients with severe pulmonary hypertension, the creation of an RLS via atrial septostomy has been shown to provide symptomatic benefit.[22–24] Nootens and colleagues[4] studied the prevalence and significance of PFO in patients with pulmonary hypertension and found no difference in the prevalence of PFO in these patients compared with the general population (25%–30%). In addition, they did not find any difference in 5-year survival or exercise tolerance.

ROLE FOR PATENT FORAMEN OVALE CLOSURE IN PATIENTS WITH CHRONIC OBSTRUCTIVE PULMONARY DISEASE

Although PFO with RLS, particularly in the presence of pulmonary hypertension, can contribute to hypoxemia in patients with COPD, it is unclear whether there is any benefit to PFO closure in this subgroup of patients. Ilkhanoff and colleagues[25] studied patients referred for percutaneous closure of a PFO at a single center. Ten patients underwent PFO closure for hypoxia; of those patients, 4 had persistent hypoxemia at rest, 6 had intermittent hypoxemia, and 2 had platypnea-orthodeoxia. The mean PAP in the group was 45 mm Hg. Of note, the patients in this study had significant pulmonary disease in the forms of sarcoid, obesity-hypoventilation syndrome, and thromboembolic lung disease. There was an improvement in the mean arterial oxygen saturation level after PFO closure (87% ± 6.5% preprocedure to 96% ± 2.9%). One patient had a transient ischemic attack (TIA) after an initially unsuccessful closure attempt. A retrospective study by Tahlawi and colleagues[26] studied the effects of PFO closure in 9 patients with chronic pulmonary disease and found no significant improvement in New York Heart Association (NYHA) functional class after PFO closure. A more recent, larger, single-center, retrospective study of PFO closure in 97 patients with chronic lung disease showed decrease in oxygen requirement and improvement in NYHA class after closure (51% of patients had improved NYHA class >1, P<.001; 34% of patients experienced a decrease in O_2 requirements, P<.001).[27] The study used contrast TTE and found that patients with a substantial RLS experienced significantly more symptom relief with PFO closure. Fenster and colleagues[27] described a 5-year single-center experience in which a large cohort of patients with chronic respiratory insufficiency underwent transcatheter PFO closure for dyspnea and hypoxia. All patients were assessed using TTE and, in those without a resting RLS, provocative maneuvers were used to elicit transseptal shunting. PFO closure was performed only if the patient had symptomatic hypoxemia, clear RLS on intracardiac echocardiography (ICE), and no significant pulmonary hypertension. Repeat saline contrast TTE was performed at 1 month and 6 months after the procedure; exercise testing, supplemental O_2 requirements, and NYHA class were assessed before and after the closure. At baseline, 54% of patients had NYHA class 3 symptoms, and 67% of the patients had coexisting pulmonary disease. Seventy-seven percent of patients had a resting shunt and an atrial septal aneurysm was present in 39% of patients. Procedural success was achieved in 99% of the patients and clinical success was observed in 70% of patients. NYHA class improvement was seen in a little more than half of the patients and 34% of patients were able to decrease their O_2 requirements. Male gender and coexisting pulmonary disease were associated with a lower rate of clinical improvement.

PATENT FORAMEN OVALE AND SLEEP APNEA

OSA is present in 24% of men and 9% of women in the general population, with increasing prevalence of this disorder caused by the increasing rates of obesity. Studies have indicated that a higher prevalence of PFO may be seen in people with OSA, with some suggesting that the prevalence may be as high as 65%.[1,28] OSA is characterized by collapse of the pharyngeal smooth muscles during exhalation resulting in airway obstruction during sleep in the recumbent position and subsequent decrease in arterial oxygen saturation. Shanoudy and colleagues[1] studied the prevalence of PFO in 48 patients with known sleep apnea and 24 control subjects. A greater proportion of patients with OSA had PFOs compared with the controls (69% vs 17%; P<.0001). The investigators also observed that the baseline oxygen saturations were similar in all patients with sleep apnea regardless of the presence or absence of a PFO (93.9% + 1.7% vs 95% + 0.6%; P = .007). However, a significantly greater decrease in O_2 saturation was noted in the PFO group compared with patients with OSA without a PFO. In another study of 78 patients with OSA and 89 without OSA,[29] TCD showed a statistically significant higher prevalence of PFO in the OSA group (27% vs 15%; P<.05). Mojadidi and colleagues[30] studied the prevalence of RLS in 100 patients with diagnosed OSA compared with 200 control subjects without OSA using TCD. They observed a much higher prevalence of RLS in patients with OSA compared with those without diagnosed sleep apnea (42% vs 19%; P<.0001). These findings suggest that OSA alters the pressure gradient across the atrial septum, which predisposes to opening of the septal foramen and increases RLS.

The prevalence of pulmonary hypertension in patients with OSA is approximately 15% to 20%.[31] The development of pulmonary hypertension can be associated with obstructive ventilation patterns, daytime hypoxemia, and hypercapnia. There are large intrathoracic pressure swings caused by forced expiration and inspiration against an obstructed upper airway. These pressure swings can lead to negative pleural pressures of up to −80 cm H_2O, and even pulsus paradoxus with leftward shift of the interatrial septum.[32] In addition, recurrent hypoxemia leads to reflex pulmonary vasoconstriction and long-standing pulmonary vasoconstriction, which in turn leads to chronic changes in pulmonary vasculature and pulmonary hypertension. Systolic transmural PAP increases acutely by 10 mm Hg or more during episodes of sleep apnea.[33] This acute effect on PAP may lead to increased RA pressure and exacerbation of RLS through a PFO. These changes in hemodynamics potentially cause greater levels of desaturation during episodes of sleep apnea. Beelke and colleagues[34] studied patients with OSA with a PFO during sleep with a TCD. These patients did not have any shunting across the PFO while awake, but significant RLS occurred during episodes of apnea while asleep. Therefore, there are multiple mechanisms that lead to increased RLS through a PFO in patients with OSA.

Pinet and colleagues[35] describe the case of a patient with OSA and a large PFO with baseline RLS in which treatment with continuous positive airway pressure for 1 week led to cessation of the baseline RLS with shunting present only during Valsalva. It has been hypothesized that recurrent episodes of sleep apnea can cause long-term hemodynamic changes resulting in increased right atrial pressures and chronic RLS.[28] There are case reports that describe improvement in sleep apnea symptoms and the number of apneic and hypopneic episodes after PFO closure in patients with OSA.[36,37] Silver and colleagues[36] reported the case of a 51-year-old man with severe OSA who underwent PFO closure following an ischemic stroke. Polysomnographic studies done before and after the PFO closure showed a clear decrease in the number of apnea episodes and the patient reported improvement in symptoms. This improvement was not explained by weight loss, medications, or changes in sleep duration and was attributed to the PFO closure. In another case, significant improvements in daytime sleepiness, fatigue, and exercise were seen in a 42-year-old man following PFO closure.[37] The mechanism underlying this improvement is unclear and, although the reduction in desaturation likely plays a role, there are potentially other unidentified mechanisms that may be responsible (Fig. 4).

PATENT FORAMEN OVALE AND PLATYPNEA-ORTHODEOXIA

POS is a rare clinical entity in which patients experience dyspnea and hypoxemia while upright, which improve in the recumbent position. Platypnea (flat breathing), first described in 1949, refers to shortness of breath in the upright position, whereas orthodeoxia refers to arterial hypoxemia that is worse with standing and made better by lying down.[38] Blood shunting through a PFO or atrial septal defect is the most common cause for this condition. Other causes include liver disease and severe pulmonary disorders.[38,39] The role of PFO closure in this disorder has been evaluated in small studies. Mojadidi and colleagues[40] examined 683 patients referred for conditions associated with PFO, of whom 17 (2.5%) had POS and underwent PFO closure. Eleven of 17 patients (65%) in whom the PFO was closed experienced improvement in hypoxemia and dyspnea in the upright position. It was noted that patients who did not experience improvement in symptoms or oxygen levels had primary lung disease with pulmonary hypertension. In another single-center study, PFO closure was evaluated in 52 patients with POS.[41] Associated conditions included pneumonectomy, ascending arch dilatation, and arch surgery, although approximately 38% of patients did not have any associated condition to explain the POS. There was a significant improvement in hypoxemia and symptoms after PFO closure. Although a residual shunt was found in 20% of patients, even those patients experienced significant relief in symptoms.

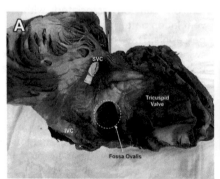
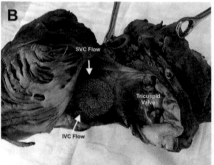

Fig. 4. (A) A large PFO within the fossa ovalis. (B) Closure device occluding the large PFO and most of the fossa so as to prevent shunting from the IVC across the septum.

POS can also develop following pneumonectomy, although this is an uncommon occurrence.[42] More common causes of dyspnea after pneumonectomy include loss of alveoli, postoperative pain, and diaphragmatic paralysis. Barkis and colleagues[42] reported the development of POS in 4 patients following pneumonectomy. The investigators highlight the importance of considering RLS through a PFO in the setting of postoperative dyspnea and low oxygen saturations along with normal radiological findings in the remaining lung. In these situations, RLS leading to systemic desaturation develops despite normal right-sided pressures, possibly because the pneumonectomy affects the cardiac position such that the PFO opens further.

PATENT FORAMEN OVALE AND PULMONARY ARTERIOVENOUS MALFORMATION

A pulmonary arteriovenous malformation (PAVM) is defined as an abnormal connection between a pulmonary artery and a pulmonary vein. The incidence in the general population is around 0.04%. This condition is associated with hereditary hemorrhagic telangiectasia in which excess vascular endothelial growth factor is thought to stimulate the growth of arteriovenous malformations. Kijima and colleagues[43] described the case of a 52-year-old man with hereditary hemorrhagic telangiectasia who presented with multiple TIAs and was found to have multiple small PAVMs, as well as a PFO. The PFO was successfully closed percutaneously using a 25-mm Gore Helex Septal Occluder (WL Gore and Associates, Inc, Flagstaff, AZ). The investigators also describe a case of a 71-year-old woman with a PFO and 2 prior strokes referred for PFO closure. Immediately after PFO closure, a large residual RLS was noted on ICE imaging. Pulmonary artery angiography revealed a large PAVM that was subsequently closed using an Amplatzer Vascular Plug IV (St. Jude Medical, St Paul, MN). These cases highlight that either a PFO or a PAVM may cause a large RLS and that both entities can coexist.

SUMMARY

A PFO is a common anatomic finding in 20% of the normal population. Although most people with a PFO are not symptomatic, significant hypoxemia can occur in circumstances in which hemodynamic or anatomic changes predispose to increased right-to-left intra-atrial shunting. The subsequent hypoxemia produces substantial dyspnea that may affect the patient's quality of life, independent of underlying pulmonary disease. Profound hypoxemia caused by right-to-left shunt across the interatrial septum usually responds to percutaneous PFO closure. An important impediment to successful treatment is the lack of awareness of the potential role of a PFO in this condition.

REFERENCES

1. Shanoudy H, Soliman A, Raggi P, et al. Prevalence of patient foramen ovale and its contribution to hypoxemia in patients with obstructive sleep apnea. Chest 1998;113:91–6.
2. Soliman A, Shanoudy H, Liu J, et al. Increased prevalence of patent foramen ovale in patients with severe chronic obstructive pulmonary disease. J Am Soc Echocardiogr 1999;12:99–105.
3. Kasper W, Geibel A, Tiede N, et al. Patent foramen ovale in patients with haemodynamically significant pulmonary embolism. Lancet 1992;340(8819):561–4.
4. Nootens MT, Berarducci LA, Kaufmann E, et al. The prevalence and significance of a patent foramen ovale in pulmonary hypertension. Chest J 1993; 104(6):1673–5.
5. Di Tullio MR, Sacco RL, Sciacca RR, et al. Patent foramen ovale and the risk of ischemic stroke in a multiethnic population. J Am Coll Cardiol 2007; 49(7):797–802.
6. Movsowitz C, Podolsky LA, Meyerowitz CB, et al. Patent foramen ovale: a nonfunctional embryological remnant or a potential cause of significant pathology? J Am Soc Echocardiogr 1992;5(3):259–70.
7. Godart F, Rey C, Prat A, et al. Atrial right-to-left shunting causing severe hypoxaemia despite normal right-sided pressures. Report of 11 consecutive cases corrected by percutaneous closure. Eur Heart J 2000;21(6):483–9.
8. Gallaher ME, Sperling DR, Gwinn JL, et al. Functional drainage of the inferior vena cava into the left atrium—three cases. Am J Cardiol 1963;12:561–6.
9. Thomas JD, Tabakin BS, Ittleman FP. Atrial septal defect with right to left shunt despite normal pulmonary artery pressure. J Am Coll Cardiol 1987;9: 221–4.
10. Dubourg O, Bourdarias JP, Farcot JC, et al. Contrast echocardiographic visualization of cough-induced right to left shunt through a patent foramen ovale. J Am Coll Cardiol 1984;4:587–94.
11. Nazzal SB, Bansal RC, Fitzmorris SJ, et al. Platypnea-orthodeoxia as a cause of unexplained hypoxemia in an 82-yr-old female. Cathet Cardiovasc Diagn 1990;19:242–5.
12. Laybourn KA, Martin ET, Cooper RAS, et al. Platypnea and orthodeoxia: shunting associated with an aortic aneurysm. J Thorac Cardiovasc Surg 1997; 113:955–6.

13. Hacievliyagil SS, Gunen H, Kosar FM, et al. Prevalence and clinical significance of a patent foramen ovale in patients with chronic obstructive pulmonary disease. Respir Med 2006;100(5):903–10.

14. Shaikh ZF, Kelly JL, Shrikrishna D, et al. Patent foramen ovale is not associated with hypoxemia in severe chronic obstructive pulmonary disease and does not impair exercise performance. Am J Respir Crit Care Med 2014;189(5):540–7.

15. Martolini D, Tanner R, Shrikrishna D, et al. Impact of a patent foramen ovale (PFO) presence in patients with GOLD stage II chronic obstructive pulmonary disease (COPD). Eur Respir J 2012;40(Suppl 56):P250.

16. Renzetti AD, McClement JH, Litt BD. The Veterans Administration cooperative study of pulmonary function. Am J Med 1966;41:115–29.

17. Jones NL, Burrows B, Fletcher CM. Serial studies of 100 patients with chronic airway obstruction in London and Chicago. Thorax 1967;22:327–34.

18. Elwing J, Panos RJ. Pulmonary hypertension associated with COPD. Int J Chronic Obstructive Pulm Dis 2008;3(1):55–70.

19. Moudgil R, Michelakis ED, Archer SL. Hypoxic pulmonary vasoconstriction. J Appl Physiol 2005; 98(1):390–403.

20. Young D, Mark H. Fate of the patient with the Eisenmenger syndrome. Am J Cardiol 1971;28: 658–69.

21. Austin GW, Morrow AG, Berry WB. Experimental studies of the surgical treatment of primary pulmonary hypertension. J Thorac Cardiovasc Surg 1964; 48:448–55.

22. Nihill MR, O'Laughlin MP, Mullins CE. Effects of atrial septostomy in patients with terminal cor pulmonale due to pulmonary vascular disease. Cathet Cardiovasc Diagn 1991;24(3):166–72.

23. Hausknecht TJ, Sims RE, Nihill MR, et al. Successful palliation of primary pulmonary hypertension by atrial septostomy. Am J Cardiol 1990;65:1045–6.

24. Collins TJ, Moore JW, Kirby WC. Atrial septostomy for pulmonary hypertension. Am Heart J 1988;116:873–4.

25. Ilkhanoff L, Naidu S, Rohtagi S, et al. Transcatheter device closure of interatrial septal defects in patients with hypoxia. J Interv Cardiol 2005;8(4):227–32.

26. El Tahlawi M, Jop B, Bonello B, et al. Should we close hypoxaemic patent foramen ovale and interatrial shunts on a systematic basis? Arch Cardiovasc Dis 2009;102(11):755–9.

27. Fenster BE, Nguyen B, Buckner JK, et al. Effectiveness of percutaneous closure of patent foramen ovale for hypoxemia. Am J Cardiol 2013;112(8):1258–62.

28. Beelke M, Angelib S, Del Setteb M, et al. Prevalence of patent foramen ovale in subjects with obstructive sleep apnea: a transcranial Doppler ultrasound study. Sleep Med 2003;4:219–23.

29. Shiomi T, Guilleminault C, Stoohs R, et al. Leftward shift of the interventricular septum and pulsus paradoxus in obstructive sleep apnea syndrome. Chest 1991;100:894–902.

30. Mojadidi MK, Bokhoor PI, Gevorgyan R, et al. Sleep apnea in patients with and without a right-to-left shunt. J Clin Sleep Med 2015;11(11):1299.

31. Brinker JA, Weiss JL, Lappe DL, et al. Leftward septal displacement during right ventricular loading in man. Circulation 1980;61:626–33.

32. Iwase N, Kikuchi Y, Hida W, et al. Effects of repetitive airway obstruction on O_2 saturation and systemic and pulmonary arterial pressure in anesthetized dogs. Am Rev Respir Dis 1992;146:1402–10.

33. Schafer H, Hasper E, Ewig S, et al. Pulmonary haemodynamics in obstructive sleep apnoea: time course and associated factors. Eur Respir J 1998; 12:679–84.

34. Beelke M, Angeli S, Del Sette M, et al. Obstructive sleep apnea can be provocative for right-to-left shunting through a patent foramen ovale. Sleep 2002;25:21–7.

35. Pinet C, Orehek J. CPAP suppression of awake right-to-left shunting through patent foramen ovale in a patient with obstructive sleep apnoea. Thorax 2005;60:880–1.

36. Silver B, Greenbaum A, McCarthy S. Improvement in sleep apnea associated with closure of a patent foramen ovale. J Clin Sleep Med 2007;3:295–6.

37. Agnoletti G, Iserin L, Lafont A, et al. Obstructive sleep apnoea and patent foramen ovale: successful treatment of symptoms by percutaneous foramen ovale closure. J Interv Cardiol 2005;18:393–5.

38. Cheng TO. Platypnea-orthodeoxia syndrome: etiology, differential diagnosis, and management. Catheter Cardiovasc Interv 1999;47:64–6.

39. Seward JB, Hayes DL, Smith HC, et al. Platypnea-orthodeoxia: clinical profile, diagnostic workup, management, and report of seven cases. Mayo Clin Proc 1984;59(4):221–31. Elsevier.

40. Mojadidi MK, Gevorgyan R, Noureddin N, et al. The effect of patent foramen ovale closure in patients with platypnea-orthodeoxia syndrome. Catheter Cardiovasc Interv 2015;86:701–7.

41. Shah AH, Osten M, Leventhal A, et al. Percutaneous intervention to treat platypnea-orthodeoxia syndrome: the Toronto experience. JACC Cardiovasc Interv 2016;9(18):1928–38.

42. Bakris NC, Siddiqi AJ, Fraser CD, et al. Right-to-left interatrial shunt after pneumonectomy. Ann Thorac Surg 1997;63(1):198–201.

43. Kijima Y, Rafique AM, Tobis JM. Patent foramen ovale combined with pulmonary arteriovenous malformation. JACC Cardiovasc Interv 2016;9(20): 2169–71, 47.

Transcatheter Closure of Patent Foramen Ovale
Devices and Technique

Matthew J. Price, MD

KEYWORDS

- Patent foramen ovale • Cryptogenic stroke • Amplatzer PFO occluder
- Amplatzer cribriform occluder • CARDIOFORM septal occluder

KEY POINTS

- A comprehensive preprocedure evaluation should be performed to exclude known mechanisms of ischemic stroke.
- Transesophageal echocardiography is critical to exclude other causes of cardiac emboli, confirm the presence of a patent foramen ovale (PFO), and define its anatomic characteristics.
- Key aspects to reduce procedural complications include performing all catheter exchanges within the left atrium over a stiff wire placed within one of the pulmonary veins and by thorough de-airing and flushing of the delivery sheath and occluder.
- Although device sizing is usually straightforward, special consideration is required in cases that have a redundant, aneurysmal interatrial septum or a thick septum secundum.
- Fastidious technique, combined with intracardiac imaging under conscious sedation, can minimize procedural complications and enhance procedural success.

INTRODUCTION

Transcatheter closure of a patent foramen ovale (PFO) reduces the risk of recurrent cryptogenic stroke compared with medical therapy.[1] However, the absolute yearly risk of recurrent stroke is quite low even in patients who are treated medically.[2] Patients undergoing PFO closure are generally young (ie, younger than 60), and any serious procedural complication can have substantial long-term implications. Furthermore, PFO closure is a prophylactic procedure, and will not provide the patient with symptomatic improvement, except in cases of hypoxemia due to right-to-left shunt or possibly migraine headaches.[3,4] Therefore, appropriate patient selection is critical, and the procedural safety is paramount. Herein, we review key characteristics of the devices currently available for transcatheter PFO closure within the United States, and highlight key technical aspects of the PFO closure procedure that will maximize procedural success.

PREPROCEDURE EVALUATION
Workup for Cryptogenic Stroke

A comprehensive preprocedure evaluation is required to exclude known mechanisms of ischemic stroke, including thromboembolism, atheroembolism from aortic or carotid disease, arterial dissection, intracranial atherosclerosis, and vasculitis (**Fig. 1**).[5] Imaging assessments include MRI or computed tomography (CT) scanning of the head to rule out small vessel disease or lacunar infarct; intracranial and extracranial imaging (MR angiography or CT angiography) to rule out atherosclerotic plaque, arterial dissection, or other vascular diseases; and transesophageal echocardiography (TEE) to rule out significant aortic atheroma or intracardiac sources of thromboemboli other than a PFO. A neurologist should formally assess the patient to confirm the diagnosis of cryptogenic stroke. In one study of patients with cryptogenic stroke, clinical features more frequent among

---

Division of Cardiovascular Diseases, Scripps Clinic, 9898 Genesee Avenue, AMP-200, La Jolla, CA 92037, USA
E-mail address: price.matthew@scrippshealth.org

Intervent Cardiol Clin 6 (2017) 555–567
http://dx.doi.org/10.1016/j.iccl.2017.05.001
2211-7458/17/© 2017 Elsevier Inc. All rights reserved.

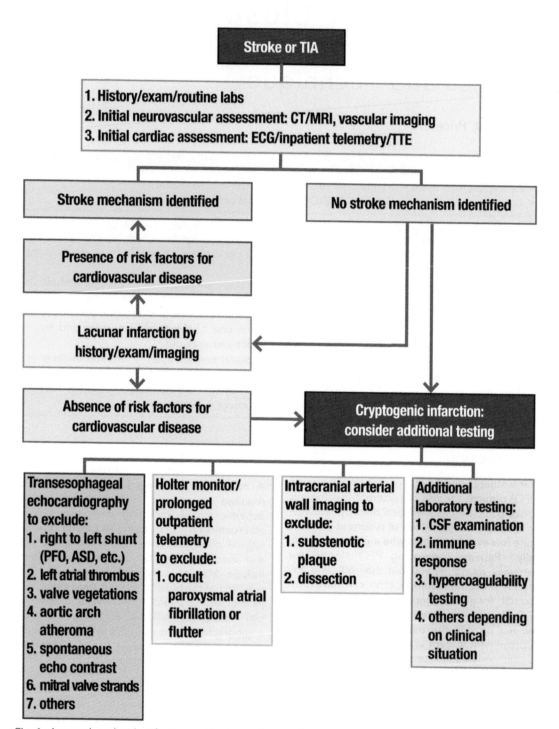

Fig. 1. Approach to the identification and further evaluation of cryptogenic stroke. CSF, cerebrospinal fluid; ECG, electrocardiogram. (*Adapted from* Yaghi S, Elkind MS. Cryptogenic stroke: a diagnostic challenge. Neurol Clin Pract 2014;4:386–93.)

patients with a PFO included a history of prolonged travel (odds ratio [OR] 8.77; 95% CI 1.78–43.3), history of deep venous thrombosis or pulmonary embolism (OR 4.39; 95% CI 1.23–15.69), Valsalva maneuver preceding the onset of focal neurologic symptoms (OR 3.33; 95% CI 1.15–9.64), history of migraine headache (OR 2.30; 95% CI 1.07–4.92), and stroke on awakening (OR 4.53; 95% CI 1.26–16.2).[6]

Anatomic Evaluation by Transesophageal Echocardiography

In addition to helping exclude other cardiac sources of stroke and confirming the presence of a PFO, TEE can provide important insight into the thromboembolic risk of the PFO and the technical approach to transcatheter closure. In the RESPECT (Randomized Evaluation of Recurrent Stroke Comparing PFO Closure to Established Standard of Care) trial, there was a trend toward particular benefit for PFO closure over medical therapy in patients with larger shunts and atrial septal aneurysm.[7] However, this has not been confirmed in meta-analyses,[1,8] and in another study, smaller shunts were associated with a higher risk of recurrent cryptogenic stroke.[9] Larger Eustachian valves also may be associated with higher thromboembolic risk, possibly by acting as a baffle directing inferior vena cava (IVC) flow toward the PFO.[10] TEE can identify a false-negative transthoracic echocardiogram bubble study, and careful inspection of blood flow within the right atrium (RA) can also identify a false-negative study on the TEE itself. During the bubble study, one should visualize the flow of bubbles to the site of the PFO; in some patients, IVC flow will shunt blood arriving from the upper arms (the site of agitated saline injection) away from the interatrial septum (IAS), resulting in an inadequate assessment of the presence of a right-to-left shunt. The presence of a floppy, aneurysmal IAS and/or a thick septum secundum (eg, due to lipomatous hypertrophy) increases the likelihood that a larger device will be required for successful closure (**Fig. 2**). In some cases, TEE demonstrates the presence of a small atrial septal defect (ASD) rather than a PFO.

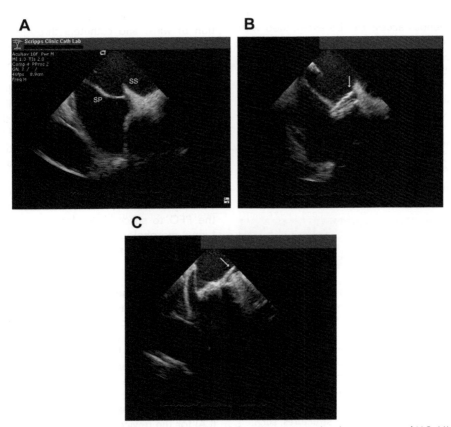

Fig. 2. Upsizing of occluder device for successful closure of a PFO associated with an aneurysmal IAS. (*A*) Baseline ICE demonstrates a wide dispersion of the IAS during the respiratory cycle; at the time of maximal dispersion, the septum primum (SP) is significantly displaced from septum secundum (SS) at the site of the PFO. (*B*) A 25-mm occluder device is implanted, but during the respiratory cycle, the left atrial disc falls below the SS into the PFO tunnel (*arrow*). This could result in a substantial residual shunt or even embolism after device release. (*C*) The initial occluder is removed and exchanged for a 30-mm device. The LA disc of this device straddles the SS (*arrow*) throughout inspiration and expiration.

Contraindications

The presence of any contraindications should be excluded before attempting PFO closure (Box 1).

PROCEDURAL APPROACH

Venous Access

The size and number of venous sheaths depend on the type of device and adjunctive imaging to be used. One venous access is required to deliver the device. A second is required to introduce the intracardiac echocardiography (ICE) catheter if that is the chosen imaging approach. Aggressive hydration with normal saline in the preoperative holding area can help reduce the time required for access, as patients are often dehydrated from being NPO (nothing by mouth).

Introducer sheath for device delivery

All sizes of the St Jude PFO and Cribiform Septal Occluders (St Jude Medical, St Paul, MN) can be delivered through an 8-Fr or 9-Fr delivery sheath. Therefore, for these devices, right femoral venous access can be established with a smaller introducer sheath (eg, 6 Fr) that can then be exchanged for the delivery sheath once a stiff wire has been placed into the left upper pulmonary vein. Alternatively, an 11-Fr introducer sheath can be placed into the right femoral vein at the beginning of the procedure, through which the 8-Fr or 9-Fr delivery sheath can be advanced. All sizes of the CARDIOFORM Septal Occluder (W.L. Gore & Associates, Inc, Flagstaff, AZ) can be introduced through an 11-Fr introducer sheath.

Box 1
Examples of contraindications to patent foramen ovale (PFO) closure

- Patients with intracardiac mass, vegetation, tumor, or thrombus at the intended site of implant, or documented evidence of venous thrombus in the vessels through which access to the PFO is gained.

- Patients whose vasculature, through which access to the PFO is gained, is inadequate to accommodate the appropriate sheath size.

- Patients with anatomy in which the device size required would interfere with other intracardiac or intravascular structures, such as valves or pulmonary veins.

- Patients with active endocarditis or other untreated infections.

Adapted from the Amplatzer PFO Occluder instructions for use.

Introducer sheath for intracardiac echocardiography

A second venous sheath is required for the ICE catheter. The ViewFlex Xtra ICE catheter (St Jude Medical) can be advanced through a 9 Fr sheath. The Accunav ICE catheter (Siemens, Malvern, PA) is available in 8 or 10 Fr. Although the 8-Fr sheath has a lower profile, the shaft is floppier and longer than the 10-Fr catheter, which can make manipulation slightly more challenging. The 10-Fr catheter can be easily advanced through an 11-Fr introducer sheath. If the operator chooses to use the left femoral vein access for the ICE catheter, a long sheath (eg, 30 cm in length) should be selected to minimize the amount of manipulation that is required to advance the ICE catheter into the IVC, which can be difficult due to venous tortuosity.

Special scenarios

As long as no thrombus is present, an IVC filter does not exclude a transcatheter approach to PFO closure. However, the amount of manipulation of wires and catheters through the filter should be minimized as much as possible. In many patients, the distal tip of a 30-cm introducer sheath placed within the right common femoral vein will extend just past the filter. Multiple passes through the filter can be eliminated by placing 2 long 11-Fr sheaths from the right femoral vein into the IVC at the start of the procedure, one for the ICE catheter and the other for the delivery sheath of any particular device that is chosen.

Some operators have advocated the use of transseptal puncture at a site separate from the PFO to successfully close cases with long tunnel morphologies (eg, >12 mm in length).[11] The results of this approach have been mixed, with some small studies demonstrating more frequent residual shunt.[12] In addition, a transseptal approach adds an incremental procedural risk of pericardial effusion and tamponade,[13] which might be considered unacceptable for a procedure that is very low risk when using standard approaches. For cases using the transseptal approach, transseptal puncture can first be performed through a transseptal sheath introduced through the right femoral vein, which then can be exchanged over a stiff wire in the left atrium (LA) for the device delivery sheath.

Patent Foramen Ovale Crossing

Intravenous unfractionated heparin is administered either before or shortly after PFO crossing for a goal activated clotting time of 250 to 300 seconds. A diagnostic multipurpose-shaped catheter (4, 5, or 6 Fr) is advanced over a standard 0.035-inch J-tipped wire to the base of the RA. In the straight anteroposterior (AP) projection, the multipurpose catheter should be rotated such that it is directed up and to the right, toward the fossa ovalis (Fig. 3A). In the setting of a reasonably sized PFO, the PFO can be crossed easily by simply advancing a standard 0.35-inch wire from this position or by making slight corrections to the path of the wire by minor counterclockwise or clockwise rotation of the multipurpose catheter from its position in the low RA. For smaller PFOs or those with stiff long tunnels, more support may be needed, and the catheter can be advanced closer to the IAS to provide more support for wire crossing. The wire even can be withdrawn to just inside the distal tip of the catheter to provide maximal stiffness, and the catheter advanced gently across the PFO with slight manipulation. Rarely the wire/and or catheter will not be able to be directed into the fossa ovalis due to RA enlargement or cardiac rotation. In this situation, ICE or TEE imaging can be helpful to direct the wire to the appropriate location.

Once the 0.35-inch J-tipped wire enters the LA, the operator should carefully advance it into the left upper pulmonary vein (LUPV). The friable and thin-walled left atrial appendage (LAA) should be assiduously avoided, as wire probing or other manipulation within this structure can cause a perforation and subsequent cardiac tamponade. The LUPV can be cannulated by clockwise (ie, posterior) rotation of the multipurpose catheter from the mid-LA with gentle probing of the wire. Fluoroscopy will demonstrate the wire going up and to the right outside of the cardiac shadow (see Fig. 3B). ICE or TEE can confirm that the wire is in the LUPV and not the LAA (Fig. 4). On occasion, the LUPV cannot be cannulated because a stiff tunnel forces the wire and catheter toward the roof of the LA. In this situation, more aggressive clockwise rotation of the catheter will direct the wire into the right upper pulmonary vein, which can then be used for wire exchange and delivery catheter advancement. Alternatively, a pig-tail–shaped wire (for example, the Protrack wire [Baylis Medical, Montreal, QC, Canada], Confida wire [Medtronic, Minneapolis MN], or Safari wire [Boston Scientific, Marlborough, MA]) can be advanced into the body of the LA for further sheath exchanges.

Once the upper pulmonary vein is cannulated, the multipurpose catheter is then advanced over the wire deep within the vein and the soft wire exchange for an Amplatz-type stiff exchange-length wire (see Fig. 3C). A stiff wire with a shorter soft tip (eg, 3 cm) is helpful, as the wire with a longer soft tip may prolapse out of the pulmonary vein and into the LA when the delivery equipment is advanced over it.

Occluder Deployment

Several types of occluders can be used to close the PFO once the wire is placed within the upper pulmonary vein. Listed in the following sections are the devices available in the United States, a brief description of their unique properties, and the technical approach to their deployment.

Amplatzer patent foramen ovale occluder

Indication. The Amplatzer PFO Occluder (St Jude Medical) is indicated for percutaneous transcatheter closure of a PFO to reduce the risk of recurrent ischemic stroke in patients, predominantly between the ages of 18 and 60 years, who have had a cryptogenic stroke due to a presumed paradoxic embolism, as determined by a neurologist and cardiologist following an evaluation to exclude known causes of ischemic stroke.

Device description. The device is a self-expanding nitinol mesh that consists of 2 discs, each with a sewn polyester patch, and a central connecting waist. Radiopaque marker bands are located on the distal and proximal ends (Fig. 5). There are 3 sizes available: 18 mm, 25 mm, and 35 mm. The device size signifies the diameter of the RA disc. For the 18-mm device, the LA disc is also 18 mm in diameter; for the 25-mm device, the LA disc is 18 mm in diameter; and for the 35-mm device, the LA disc is 25 mm in diameter. The occluder is delivered through a dedicated sheath using a delivery cable that is attached to the proximal end of the occluder via an end screw. The 18-mm and 25-mm occluders can be delivered through an 8-Fr delivery sheath, whereas the 35-mm device requires a 9-Fr delivery sheath.

Device sizing. The PFO Occluder instructions for use describe a sizing algorithm based on the lesser of the distance from the PFO to the aortic root and the distance from the PFO to the superior vena cava orifice as determined by the short and long axes of the IAS visualized by TEE or ICE. An 18-mm, 25-mm, and 35-mm device is recommended if the distance is 9.0 to 12.4 mm, 12.5 to 17.4 mm, or ≥17.5 mm, respectively. If the distance is <9.0 mm, it is not recommended to implant a device. In cases in which an atrial septal aneurysm is present, a

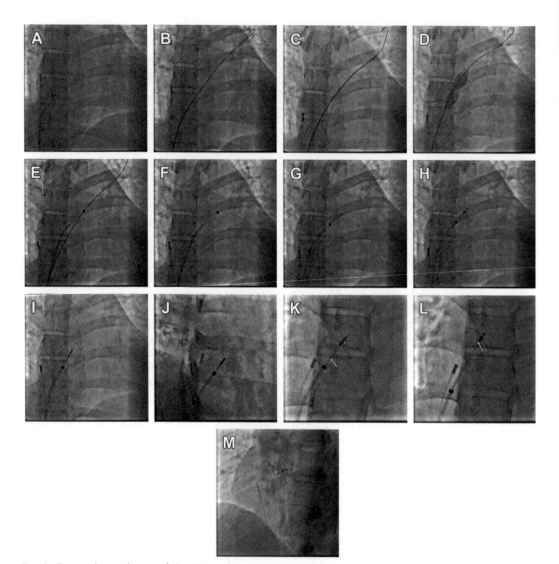

Fig. 3. Transcatheter closure of the PFO with a CARDIOFORM Septal Occluder. (A) A multipurpose (MP) diagnostic catheter (either 5-Fr or 6-Fr) is advanced over the wire to the base of the RA. The catheter is directed toward the IAS, a maneuver that can be assisted by aligning the orientation of the MP catheter with the direction of the imaging element of the ICE catheter. (B) A standard 0.035-inch J-tipped wire is advanced through the MP catheter across the PFO and into the LUPV. If the operator has trouble locating the PFO, ICE imaging can help to direct the wire into the fossa ovalis. In the case of small PFOs, the MP catheter can be advanced over the wire to the IAS to provide backup support for wire crossing, or even can be used to cross the PFO with the wire just inside the tip of the catheter. It is critical to place the 0.035-inch wire into the pulmonary vein, rather than the LAA, to avoid cardiac perforation and tamponade. If the wire enters the LAA rather than the LUPV, the operator can advance the MP into the mid- LA, withdraw the wire, clock the catheter (posterior rotation), and re-advance the wire; in the AP projection, the wire should go up and to the right and outside of the cardiac silhouette. (C) The MP is advanced over the 0.035-inch J-wire into the pulmonary vein, and the wire then exchanged for a 0.035-inch extra-stiff Amplatz wire, preferably with a short flexible tip (ie, 3 cm). The stiff wire will provide support for the sizing balloon (if desired) and for the delivery sheath. (D) In this case, a sizing balloon was advanced over the wire and inflated with dilute contrast, demonstrating a stretched diameter of 9 mm. (E) A 25-mm CARDIOFORM Septal Occluder delivery system is advanced over the stiff wire into the mid-LA. In general, the right side of the vertebral bodies is a rough marker for the fluoroscopic location of the PFO; a still-frame of the inflated sizing balloon also can act as a roadmap for the operator. (F) The 0.035-inch wire is withdrawn from the delivery system. (G) The distal tip of the CARDIO-FORM occluder is exposed by pushing the slider on the handle from right to left. The operator should take care that the distal tip does not interact with the far LA wall or the LAA; to avoid this, the entire system is withdrawn while pushing the slider to the left, exposing the tip but without advancing it deeper into the LA. (H) The LA disc is fully formed by pushing the actuator up and continuing to slide it to the left, until the disc is flat and the

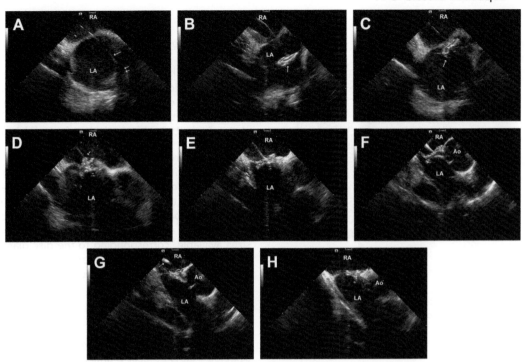

Fig. 4. ICE guidance of transcatheter PFO closure with the CARDIOFORM device. (A) The 0.035-inch guidewire (arrow) has been advanced from the RA through the PFO and into the LUPV (double arrow). (B) The left atrial disc (arrow) of the device has been formed in the mid-LA. (C) The entire system is withdrawn until the LA disc (arrow) is juxtaposed to the IAS. (D) The RA disc begins to form on the right side of the septum (arrow). (E) The right atrial disc is completely formed, and it is clear on ICE that both discs are on their respective sides of the IAS, the right atrial disc extends over the SS covering the PFO entry, and the SP is in between the 2 discs. (F) The short axis view of the atrium confirms the appropriate position of the implant, demonstrating the anterior aspects of the 2 discs straddling the SS. Ao, aorta. (G) The device is now locked, and tension is relieved as the device is connected to the delivery catheter by only the retrieval cord. The device separates from the delivery catheter (arrow) and now aligns more naturally with the axis of the IAS. (H) Final result after suture retrieval cord is withdrawn.

larger device might be considered to cover the aneurysm.

Some operators use balloon sizing to help determine device size, rather than the algorithm described in the instructions for use. With this approach, a sizing balloon is advanced across the PFO and slowly inflated with dilute contrast until a waist is visualized (see Fig. 3D). In the case of a stiff long tunnel, gentle retraction of the inflated sizing balloon can evert or open the tunnel, which might improve the final orientation of the implanted device. A device is selected that is at least 2 times the diameter of the waist of the sizing balloon. A larger size might be considered if the septum secundum is particularly thick or if there is a large atrial septal aneurysm. Many operators do not perform balloon sizing at all, and select a 25-mm occluder as the default size, but will upsize if the septum secundum is thick or an atrial septal aneurysm is present.

Device implantation. The operator advances the appropriately sized delivery sheath into the LA over the stiff wire that had been placed into the LUPV. The operator removes the wire and carefully de-airs and flushes the sheath. The operator securely attaches the proximal end of

remaining portion of the device (the RA disc) is still collapsed within the delivery catheter. (I) The entire system is withdrawn to the IAS until resistance is felt (or ICE demonstrates close proximity to the IAS), and the operator slides the actuator fully to the left and down, forming the RA disc on the right side of the IAS. (J) The RAO-caudal projection can be used to demonstrate symmetric and appropriate formation of the 2 discs. (K) Implanted CARDIOFORM device, before locking. Arrow denotes the locking loop that is confined within the delivery catheter. (L) CARDIOFORM device after locking. Note the locking loop (arrow). (M) Final result after removal of retrieval cord (left anterior oblique projection).

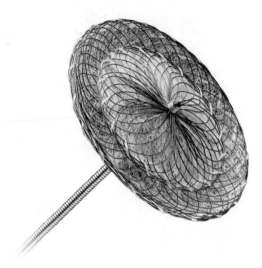

Fig. 5. The Amplatzer PFO Occluder. The device is a self-expanding nitinol mesh that consists of 2 discs, each with a sewn polyester patch, and a central connecting waist. Device size is defined by the diameter of the right atrial disc. The left atrial disc is slightly smaller than the right atrial disc, except for the 18-mm occluder, in which case both discs are identical. (*Courtesy of* St. Jude Medical, Inc, St Paul, MN; with permission.)

the PFO Occluder to the delivery cable by clockwise rotation and loads the device into the introducer, carefully flushes it, and then advances it through the delivery sheath by pushing the delivery cable. The operator pushes the delivery cable forward until the LA disc is formed in the LA, and then withdraws the sheath and device en bloc until the LA disc is adjacent to the IAS (Fig. 6A). The operator then withdraws the delivery sheath over the delivery cable, exposing the RA disc (see Fig. 6B); once the RA disc is fully exposed, the operator forms the RA disc by pushing forward on the cable (see Fig. 6C). Appropriate device position is confirmed by fluoroscopy in the left anterior oblique projection and by either ICE or TEE. A tug test can be helpful to confirm device stability. The LA and RA discs should be on their respective sides of the IAS; in particular, the LA disc should not slip off the septum secundum into the PFO tunnel. On fluoroscopy, there should be clear separation of 2 discs in the left anterior oblique projection. If the position is not satisfactory, the device can be easily retrieved by advancing the delivery sheath while retracting the delivery cable. If the position is acceptable, the operator releases the device by rotating the delivery cable counterclockwise (see Fig. 6D). Imaging guidance of PFO Occluder implantation using ICE is illustrated in Fig. 7.

Amplatzer multifenestrated (cribiform) septal occluder

Indication. The Amplatzer cribriform occluder (St Jude Medical, St Paul, MN) is intended for the closure of multifenestrated (cribriform) ASDs. Use of this device for transcatheter PFO closure in the United States is therefore off-label.

Device description. The device is a self-expanding nitinol mesh that consists of 2 discs with identical diameters, each with a sewn polyester patch, and a central connecting waist (Fig. 8). Radiopaque marker bands are located on the distal and proximal ends. There are 4 sizes available, corresponding to the disc diameter: 18 mm, 25 mm, 30 mm, and 35 mm. The 3 smaller sizes require a minimum 8-Fr delivery sheath, and the largest size requires a 9-Fr sheath.

Device size selection. Device size selection is similar to the PFO Occluder device. A device is selected that is at least 2 times the diameter of the waist of the sizing balloon. A larger size might be selected if the septum secundum is particularly thick or if there is a large atrial septal aneurysm. Alternatively, many operators do not perform balloon sizing, and choose a 25-mm occluder as the default size but will upsize if the septum secundum is thick or if an atrial septal aneurysm is present.

Device implantation. Device implantation is similar to that for the PFO Occluder. A case of ICE-guided implantation of a Cribiform Septal Occluder for transcatheter PFO closure is illustrated in Fig. 9.

CARDIOFORM septal occluder

Indication. The CARDIOFORM Septal Occluder (W.L. Gore & Associates) is indicated for the percutaneous, transcatheter closure of ostium secundum ASDs, and its use for transcatheter PFO closure is currently off-label in the United States. This safety and efficacy of this device for PFO closure is being studied in the GORE HELEX Septal Occluder/GORE Septal Occluder and Antiplatelet Medical Management for Reduction of Recurrent Stroke or Imaging-Confirmed TIA in Patients With Patent Foramen Ovale (REDUCE) clinical trial (clinicaltrials.gov identifier NCT00738894).

Device description. The CARDIOFORM Septal Occluder consists of a platinum-filled nitinol wire frame covered with expanded polytetrafluoroethylene that when fully deployed assumes a double-disc shape in which each disc has an

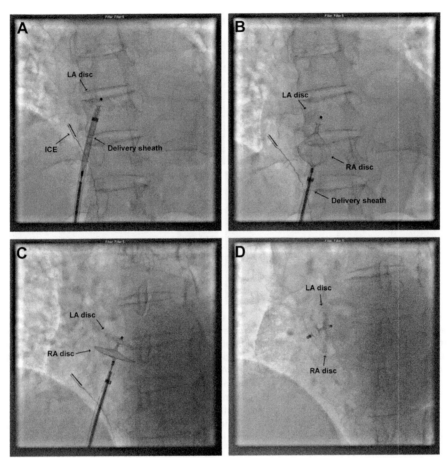

Fig. 6. Transcatheter PFO closure with a PFO Occluder. (*A*) The 8 Fr TorqueView 45° delivery sheath has been advanced from the right femoral vein into the LA. An Amplatzer PFO Occluder 25-mm device is advanced through the sheath until the LA disc is formed with the LA and the system withdrawn until the LA disc is abutting the IAS. For echocardiographic guidance, the ICE catheter is rotated clockwise, flexed posteriorly and slight to the left, and therefore points up and to the left on this AP fluoroscopic projection. (*B*) The delivery sheath is withdrawn while maintaining position of the delivery cable, exposing the RA disc. Tension from the delivery cable elongates the RA disc. (*C*) The delivery cable is now pushed forward, relieving the tension on the RA disc. The LA and RA discs are separated and slightly splayed, consistent with capture of the IAS, which is confirmed by ICE. (*D*) The device is released by counterclockwise rotation of the delivery cable. The device shifts fluoroscopic position as the tension from the delivery cable is completely relieved.

identical diameter (**Fig. 10**). There are 3 eyelets made of wound nitinol, the RA eyelet, a central eyelet, and an LA eyelet, and a locking loop that keeps the eyelets together. The occluder comes preloaded within a delivery system that consists of a 75-cm 10-Fr outer diameter rapid-exchange delivery catheter that is coupled to a handle. The delivery catheter can be advanced over a 0.035-inch (or smaller) guidewire. The operator actuates the handle to load, deploy, and lock the occluder, as well as to reposition or retrieve the occluder if necessary. A retrieval cord allows the occluder to be recaptured even after locking. The occluder is sized by the diameter of the discs. There are 4 sizes commercially available: 15, 20, 25, and 30 mm. The system can be delivered through an 11-Fr introducer sheath in the femoral vein.

Device size selection. If balloon sizing is performed, a device at least 1.8 times the waist diameter is chosen. If the septum secundum is particularly thick, and the device size based on balloon waist diameter is near the threshold for a higher size, one might consider upsizing 1 size so that the LA disc straddles the septum secundum securely and does not fall into the PFO tunnel (see **Fig. 2**). Many operators do not balloon size and choose the 25-mm size by default. Because the compressive forces

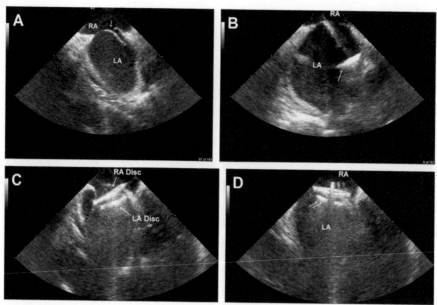

Fig. 7. ICE guidance of transcatheter PFO closure with the St Jude PFO Occluder. (*A*) The short axis of the IAS demonstrates a long, tunneled PFO. Arrow, right-sided entry into PFO. (*B*) After the delivery sheath is introduced over a wire through the PFO, the device is advanced through the sheath and then the sheath is withdrawn over the delivery cable and the LA disc of the device (*arrow*) is exposed. (*C*) After withdrawing the entire system to the IAS, the RA disc is unsheathed. ICE demonstrates that the LA and RA discs have captured the IAS. Tension from the delivery cable pulls the device toward the inferior venae cavae, which causes the device to tilt within the IAS and indent the thin tissue of the inferior-posterior septum. This image corresponds to the fluoroscopic image illustrated in Fig. 6C. (*D*) PFO occluder device after release from delivery cable. Note the smaller LA disc (*double arrow*), and the improved orientation of the device with the IAS after resolution of tension from the delivery cable. This image corresponds to the fluoroscopic image seen in Fig. 6D.

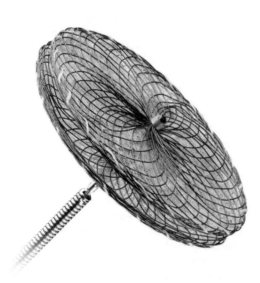

Fig. 8. The Amplatzer Multifenestrated (Cribiform) Occluder. The device is a self-expanding nitinol mesh that consists of 2 discs with identical diameters, each with a sewn polyester patch, and a central connecting waist.

between the 2 discs of the CARDIOFORM device do not differ greatly across sizes (unlike the prior generation Helex device), there is little upside to choosing a device size smaller than 25 mm even for closure of small PFOs (ie, sizing balloon waist diameter ≤10 mm).

Device implantation. The selected device delivery system must first be flushed and loaded. The occluder and catheter tip are submerged in heparinized saline and the delivery catheter flushed until air no longer exits the tip. The occluder is then loaded into the catheter by sliding the actuator knob on the handle fully from the right to the left. The catheter should then be flushed again until there are no longer any air bubbles exiting the distal tip of the catheter.

The delivery system is next advanced across the PFO and into the mid-LA over the stiff guidewire that has already been placed in the pulmonary vein (see Fig. 3E). Once the delivery sheath is in the LA, the guidewire is removed (see Fig. 3F). The operator begins to deploy the left disc of the occluder by pushing the slider

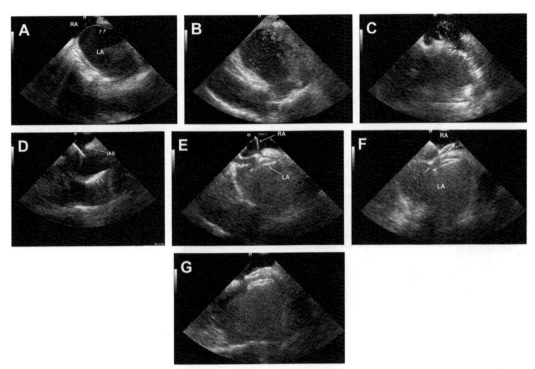

Fig. 9. ICE guidance of transcatheter PFO closure with St Jude Cribiform Septal Occluder. (*A*) Long axis of the LA demonstrates the fossa ovalis and the PFO (*double arrows*). (*B*) Agitated saline injection ("bubble study") from the femoral venous sheath demonstrates large right-to-left shunt through PFO (*arrow*). (*C*) Sizing balloon inflation demonstrates stiff tunnel (*arrows*) with a stretched diameter of approximately 11 mm. (*D*) The LA disc (*double arrows*) is exposed within the LA. Single arrow, IAS. (*E*) After the system is withdrawn to the IAS, the sheath is further withdrawn and the RA disc begins to form. (*F*) The RA disc is now fully formed, and the 2 discs capture the IAS. Tension toward the IVC by the delivery cable (*green arrow*) lifts the superior aspect of the RA disc away from the SS (*blue arrow*) and pushes the inferior aspect of the RA disc into the SP (*yellow arrow*). (*G*) Final result after release from delivery cable.

to the left. When the occluder first exits the catheter, its tip is quite rigid. Therefore, to avoid engaging the LA roof or LA appendage with the rigid end of the device, it can be helpful to withdraw the catheter over the occluder when the tip of the occluder reaches the tip of the catheter on fluoroscopy (ie, rather than continue to push the slider to the left, fix the slider with the right hand and withdraw the catheter/handle with the left hand until the slider can no longer move) (see **Fig. 3**G). Next, the operator pushes the slider up and to the left to form the LA disc. The slider should be pushed to the left until the LA disc is flat (see **Fig. 3**H). At this point, the catheter and handle are retracted en bloc until the LA disc abuts the IAS (by ICE or TEE). In the setting of a stiff, long PFO tunnel, the catheter should be withdrawn until there is tension on the disc, manifested by concave tenting of the disc on fluoroscopy. Continuing to push the slider to the left until it stops, and then down, forms the RA disc (see **Fig. 3**I).

The position and stability of the occluder should be assessed by fluoroscopy and ICE/TEE. In the fluoroscopic left anterior oblique projection, the discs should clearly be separated from one another, with slight splaying of the discs around the aorta; in the right anterior oblique caudal projection, symmetric flowering petals confirms that the 2 discs are appropriately formed (see **Fig. 3**J). ICE or TEE should demonstrate that the LA disc straddles the septum secundum and does not fall within the PFO tunnel (see **Figs. 2** and **4**). If the disc positions or shapes are unacceptable, simply pushing the slider up and to the right will recapture the discs and pushing the slider to the left will reform them.

The device is locked once position and stability are confirmed. First, the operator should hold and fix the handle with his or her right hand, making sure that there is no tension on the occluder. The operator then squeezes and slides the occluder lock (located at the distal end of the handle) to the right. This liberates the loop-shaped end

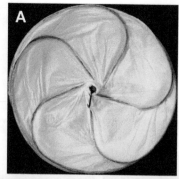

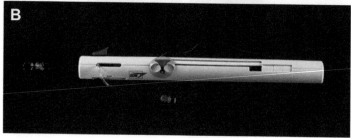

Fig. 10. CARDIOFORM Septal Occluder. This device consists of a platinum-filled nitinol wire frame covered with expanded polytetrafluoroethylene that when fully deployed assumes a double-disc shape in which each disc has an identical diameter. The delivery system consists of the (A) occluder device and delivery catheter, and (B) the handle. (*Courtesy of* Gore Medical, Inc, Flagstaff, AZ; with permission.)

of nitinol from the delivery system, which will prevent the discs from separating. Full deployment of the locking loop can be confirmed by cineangiography (see Fig. 3K, L); furthermore, the delivery catheter should fall slightly away from the occluder, as it is no longer attached to the occluder by a rigid member but rather by the delivery retrieval cord. Rarely, the locking loop may not be fully released; this can be identified by cineangiography. When this occurs, the Luer lock proximal to the handle can be unscrewed and the catheter advanced forward slightly to liberate the locking loop.

If the occluder position is unacceptable after locking, the occluder can still be retrieved, as the handle is connected to the RA eyelet by a retrieval cord. The operator withdraws the handle and catheter en bloc into the low RA to permit the locking loop to fully extend. The operator then unscrews the delivery catheter's Luer lock and withdraws the handle slowly while advancing the catheter as needed, thereby recapturing the occluder within the delivery catheter. It is important to ensure that the locking loop and eyelets to do not get caught on the distal tip of the catheter as the handle is withdrawn, as that could result in snapping of the retrieval cord.

Once the lock is deployed and the device position is acceptable, the retrieval cord is withdrawn by pulling up on the red retrieval cord lock while fixing the handle, and pulling the cord gently until it is completely removed from the handle (see Fig. 3M).

PROCEDURAL IMAGING

The transcatheter PFO closure procedure can be guided by ICE or by TEE. Although the ICE catheter increases procedural cost, ICE guidance has several advantages by obviating the need for an anesthesiologist and echocardiographer. The ICE catheter is advanced into the low-RA to mid-RA and rotated to the "home view," in which the tricuspid valve, right ventricular outflow track, and pulmonic valve are all clearly seen. The catheter is then slowly rotated clockwise. First, the mitral valve and LAA will be visualized. The catheter should then be rotated further clockwise until the mitral valve disappears from view; at this point, the catheter tip is angled posteriorly and slightly to the left. This will demonstrate the long axis of the IAS (similar to a bicaval view on TEE) (see Fig. 9A). Further clockwise rotation of the catheter by approximately 90° will then demonstrate the IAS in short axis (see Fig. 7A).

PROCEDURAL AND DEVICE-RELATED COMPLICATIONS

Transcatheter PFO closure is associated with a very low risk of procedural complications. In the RESPECT trial, device or procedure-related adverse events occurred in 22 of 499 patients (4.2%) in the closure group. The rates of procedure-related atrial fibrillation, tamponade, or cardiac thrombus were very low (0.2%,

0.4%, 0.4%, and 0.4%, respectively). Vascular complications occurred in 3 patients (0.6%). There were no cases of device embolization or intraprocedural stroke. Device-related perforation (ie, erosion) did not occur in any patients at a mean follow-up of 6.3 years (3141 patient-years).[7] There were no serious procedure-related or device-related adverse events at 6-month follow-up among the 50 patients enrolled in the nonrandomized pivotal study of the CARDIOFORM Septal Occluder for trans-catheter ASD closure (CARDIOFORM package insert). In a study of 60 consecutive patients undergoing transcatheter PFO closure with the CARDIOFORM Septal Occluder, stroke, thrombus formation, and atrial fibrillation/flutter occurred in 1 (1.7%), 1 (1.7%), and 5 (8.3%) patients, respectively.[14]

Procedural safety of transcatheter PFO closure can be maximized by using ultrasound guidance to cannulate the femoral veins; performing all catheter exchanges within the LA over a stiff wire placed in one of the pulmonary veins, or over a pig-tail–shaped wire (eg, an Inouye-type wire); by thorough de-airing and flushing of the delivery sheath and occluder to prevent air emboli during deployment, which can result in stroke, chest pain, ST-elevation, or myocardial infarction, usually involving the right coronary artery; in the case of the CARDIO-FORM device, by unsheathing the distal tip of the occluder by withdrawing the sheath while fixing the slider, thereby preventing cardiac perforation by the distal rigid member; and by appropriate device sizing and placement.

SUMMARY

Transcatheter PFO closure is a straightforward, safe procedure that in randomized clinical trials reduces the risk of recurrent cryptogenic stroke. Several occluder devices are available in the United States that can successfully close a PFO in an on-label or off-label fashion. Fastidious technique, combined with intracardiac imaging under conscious sedation, can minimize procedural complications and enhance procedural success.

REFERENCES

1. Kent DM, Dahabreh IJ, Ruthazer R, et al. Device closure of patent foramen ovale after stroke: pooled analysis of completed randomized trials. J Am Coll Cardiol 2016;67:907–17.

2. Kent DM, Ruthazer R, Weimar C, et al. An index to identify stroke-related vs incidental patent foramen ovale in cryptogenic stroke. Neurology 2013;81: 619–25.

3. Mattle HP, Evers S, Hildick-Smith D, et al. Percutaneous closure of patent foramen ovale in migraine with aura, a randomized controlled trial. Eur Heart J 2016;37:2029–36.

4. Shah AH, Osten M, Leventhal A, et al. Percutaneous intervention to treat platypnea-orthodeoxia syndrome: the Toronto experience. JACC Cardiovasc Interv 2016;9:1928–38.

5. Yaghi S, Elkind MS. Cryptogenic stroke: a diagnostic challenge. Neurol Clin Pract 2014;4:386–93.

6. Ozdemir AO, Tamayo A, Munoz C, et al. Cryptogenic stroke and patent foramen ovale: clinical clues to paradoxical embolism. J Neurol Sci 2008; 275:121–7.

7. Carroll JD, Saver JL, Thaler DE, et al. Closure of patent foramen ovale versus medical therapy after cryptogenic stroke. N Engl J Med 2013;368:1092–100.

8. Wessler BS, Thaler DE, Ruthazer R, et al. Transesophageal echocardiography in cryptogenic stroke and patent foramen ovale: analysis of putative high-risk features from the risk of paradoxical embolism database. Circ Cardiovasc Imaging 2014;7: 125–31.

9. Thaler DE, Ruthazer R, Weimar C, et al. Recurrent stroke predictors differ in medically treated patients with pathogenic vs. other PFOs. Neurology 2014;83:221–6.

10. Vale TA, Newton JD, Orchard E, et al. Prominence of the Eustachian valve in paradoxical embolism. Eur J Echocardiogr 2011;12:33–6.

11. McMahon CJ, El Said HG, Mullins CE. Use of the transseptal puncture in transcatheter closure of long tunnel-type patent foramen ovale. Heart 2002;88:E3.

12. Moon J, Kang WC, Kim S, et al. Comparison of outcomes after device closure with transseptal puncture and standard technique in patients with patent foramen ovale and ischemic events. J Interv Cardiol 2016;29:400–5.

13. Thompson AJ, Hagler DJ, Taggart NW. Transseptal puncture to facilitate device closure of "long-tunnel" patent foramen ovale. Catheter Cardiovasc Interv 2015;85:1053–7.

14. Knerr M, Bertog S, Vaskelyte L, et al. Results of percutaneous closure of patent foramen ovale with the GORE((R)) septal occluder. Catheter Cardiovasc Interv 2014;83:1144–51.

Moving?

Make sure your subscription moves with you!

To notify us of your new address, find your **Clinics Account Number** (located on your mailing label above your name), and contact customer service at:

Email: journalscustomerservice-usa@elsevier.com

800-654-2452 (subscribers in the U.S. & Canada)
314-447-8871 (subscribers outside of the U.S. & Canada)

Fax number: 314-447-8029

Elsevier Health Sciences Division
Subscription Customer Service
3251 Riverport Lane
Maryland Heights, MO 63043

*To ensure uninterrupted delivery of your subscription, please notify us at least 4 weeks in advance of move.

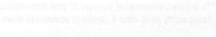

Printed and bound by CPI Group (UK) Ltd, Croydon, CR0 4YY

03/10/2024

01040383-0006